SKILLS PERFORMANCE CHECKLISTS

to accompany

Elkin, Perry, and Potter's

NURSING INTERVENTIONS & CLINICAL SKILLS

THIRD EDITION

Patricia A. Castaldi, RN, BSN, MSN

Director
Practical Nursing Program
Union County College
Plainfield, New Jersey

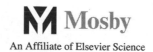
Mosby

An Affiliate of Elsevier Science

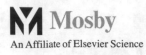

Mosby

An Affiliate of Elsevier Science

11830 Westline Industrial Drive
St. Louis, Missouri 63146

Notice

Nursing is an ever-changing field. Standard safety precautions must be followed, but as new research and clinical experience broaden our knowledge, changes in treatment and drug therapy may become necessary or appropriate. Readers are advised to check the most current product information provided by the manufacturer of each drug to be administered to verify the recommended dose, the method and duration of administration, and contraindications. It is the responsibility of the licensed prescriber, relying on experience and knowledge of the patient, to determine dosages and the best treatment for each individual patient. Neither the publisher nor the author assumes any liability for any injury and/or damage to persons or property arising from this publication.

Previous edition copyrighted 1996.

International Standard Book Number 0-323-02200-6

Executive Editor: Susan R. Epstein
Developmental Editor: Robyn L. Brinks
Publishing Services Manager: Gayle May
Project Manager: Stephanie M. Hebenstreit
Designer: Kathi Gosche

Printed in the United States of America.

Last digit is the print number: 9   8   7   6   5   4   3   2   1

Introduction to Students

The checklists in this book were developed to assist your instructors in evaluating your competence in performing the nursing interventions presented in the text *Nursing Interventions and Clinical Skills,* Third Edition. Instructors can check "Satisfactory," "Unsatisfactory," or "Needs Practice" for each step. Specific instructions or feedback can be provided in the "Comments" column. These checklists are perforated, so you can easily remove them and turn them in as required.

These checklists have been streamlined to include **only** the critical steps needed to satisfactorily master the skill. They are **not** intended to replace the text, which describes and illustrates each nursing skill in detail.

For all nursing interventions, the nurse should:

1. **Assess the client's health status** by interviewing the client, conducting a physical assessment, and reviewing the client's record.
2. **Develop a nursing diagnosis** to reflect actual or potential health concerns.
3. **Plan** by identifying goals and expected outcomes.
4. **Implement** the plan of care individualized to the client's needs.
5. **Evaluate** by determining whether goals and expected outcomes were met and observing for changes in the client's response.

Table of Contents

Performance Checklist: Skill 1.1

Standard Protocols for All Nursing Interventions

		S	U	NP	Comments

Before the Skill

1. Verify nursing intervention using physician's order or nursing care plan

2. Identify client (arm band and state name).

3. Introduce yourself to client.

4. Explain procedure and rationale.

5. Assess client's current health status and possible contraindications to specific intervention.

6. Gather appropriate equipment.

7. Perform hand hygiene for at least 10 to 15 seconds.

Nurse Alert: Manufacturers of antiseptic hand disinfectants may recommend duration for hand hygiene.

8. Adjust bed height and side rails.

9. Provide privacy for client.

During the Skill

10. Promote client involvement if possible.

11. Assess client's tolerance.

Completion Protocol

12. Ensure client's comfort and safety.

13. Raise side rails and lower bed.

14. Store or dispose of equipment properly.

15. Perform hand hygiene for at least 10 to 15 seconds.

16. Report and record nursing intervention and client's response to the procedure.

Name _____ Date _____ Instructor's Name _____

Performance Checklist: Skill 1.2

Recording

	S	U	NP	Comments

Assessment

1. Review assessments, goals, and expected outcomes, interventions, and client responses directly after client contact. ___ ___ ___ _____

Implementation

1. Identify type of documentation method(s) used by agency. ___ ___ ___ _____

2. Identify information that needs to be documented including abnormal findings, status changes, new problems or concerns, nursing actions, client response, and to whom reported. ___ ___ ___ _____

3. Document in a timely fashion. ___ ___ ___ _____

4. Determine the most effective way to document significant changes.
   a. Be factual and objective. ___ ___ ___ _____
   b. Include subjective and objective data (avoid *good, adequate, fair*, etc.). ___ ___ ___ _____
   c. Identify nursing actions taken. ___ ___ ___ _____
   d. Include client responses. ___ ___ ___ _____
   e. Identify additional plans to be implemented. ___ ___ ___ _____
   f. Specify to whom information has been reported. ___ ___ ___ _____

5. Sign or initial all written documentation. ___ ___ ___ _____

Performance Checklist: Skill 1.3

Giving a Change-of-Shift Report

	S	U	NP	Comments

Assessment

1. Gather all relevant information on client's status.   ____ ____ ____ _____

Implementation

1. Deliver report in an organized manner, describing client's needs and concerns.   ____ ____ ____ _____

2. Include pertinent information for each client.
   a. Background   ____ ____ ____ _____
   b. Assessment data   ____ ____ ____ _____
   c. Nursing diagnoses   ____ ____ ____ _____
   d. Interventions and evaluation of response
      (1) Medications and treatments, lab results, and client's response   ____ ____ ____ _____
      (2) Client teaching   ____ ____ ____ _____
   e. Family information   ____ ____ ____ _____
   f. Discharge plan   ____ ____ ____ _____
   g. Current priorities   ____ ____ ____ _____

Evaluation

1. Ask staff from oncoming shift if there are questions about report.   ____ ____ ____ _____

2. Self-evaluate tape-recorded reports for their ability to be understood.   ____ ____ ____ _____

Performance Checklist: Skill 1.4

Writing an Incident Report

	S	U	NP	Comments

Assessment

1. Use critical thinking skills to determine factors that may have contributed to incident. ____ ____ ____ _____

2. Assess and attend to safety and comfort needs of client or other individuals involved in incident. ____ ____ ____ _____

Implementation

1. Complete incident report accurately and in a timely manner. ____ ____ ____ _____

2. Use objective descriptions of what was observed. ____ ____ ____ _____

3. Describe measures implemented by caregivers at time of incident. Include times, names of witnesses, condition of individual involved, and who was notified. ____ ____ ____ _____

4. Sign written reports and obtain any additional signatures as required by agency. ____ ____ ____ _____

5. Document related observations and interventions on client's medical record. ____ ____ ____ _____

Evaluation

1. Identify actions that may prevent similar occurrences. ____ ____ ____ _____

Name _____ Date _____ Instructor's Name _____

Performance Checklist: Skill 2.1

Establishing Therapeutic Communication

	S	U	NP	Comments

Assessment

1. Determine client's need to communicate. _____ _____ _____ _____

2. Assess client's reason for seeking health care. _____ _____ _____ _____

3. Assess factors about self and client that may influence communication. _____ _____ _____ _____

4. Assess client's language and ability to speak (expressive or receptive aphasia). _____ _____ _____ _____

5. Observe client's pattern of verbal and nonverbal communication. _____ _____ _____ _____

6. Encourage client to ask for clarification during communication. _____ _____ _____ _____

Implementation

1. Use Standard Protocol. _____ _____ _____ _____

2. Create a climate of warmth and acceptance. _____ _____ _____ _____

3. Address client by name and introduce self by name and role. _____ _____ _____ _____

4. Be aware of nonverbal cues both sent and received. _____ _____ _____ _____

5. Explain purpose of interaction. _____ _____ _____ _____

6. Encourage client to seek clarification during interaction. _____ _____ _____ _____

7. Use questions appropriately.
   a. Ask one at a time. _____ _____ _____ _____
   b. Allow time to answer. _____ _____ _____ _____
   c. Use open questions. _____ _____ _____ _____
   d. Use closed questions. _____ _____ _____ _____
   e. Avoid *why?* questions. _____ _____ _____ _____

8. Use clear and concise statements. _____ _____ _____ _____

9. Focus on understanding the client, providing feedback, assisting problem solving, and providing an atmosphere of warmth and acceptance. _____ _____ _____ _____

10. Adjust time allowed based on client's needs. _____ _____ _____ _____

	S	U	NP	Comments

11. Be aware of cultural, age, and gender differences. Be alert to literacy status. ____ ____ ____ _____

12. Summarize what was discussed. Request feedback from the client. ____ ____ ____ _____

13. Use Completion Protocol. ____ ____ ____ _____

Evaluation

1. Observe responses toward communication. ____ ____ ____ _____
2. Ask client for feedback. ____ ____ ____ _____
3. Verify if information obtained is accurate. ____ ____ ____ _____

- Identify unexpected outcomes and intervene as necessary. ____ ____ ____ _____

- Record and report intervention and client's response. ____ ____ ____ _____

Performance Checklist: Skill 2.2

Comforting

	S	U	NP	Comments

Assessment

1. Observe interactions between client and others in the environment. ____ ____ ____ _____

2. Identify medications that may alter speech. ____ ____ ____ _____

3. Identify client's body language. ____ ____ ____ _____

Implementation

1. Use Standard Protocol. ____ ____ ____ _____

2. Provide a private, quiet, and calm environment. ____ ____ ____ _____

3. Respond to client's physical discomfort. ____ ____ ____ _____

4. Convey interest using eye contact and open body posture. ____ ____ ____ _____

5. Convey acceptance without judgment. ____ ____ ____ _____

6. Provide empathy. ____ ____ ____ _____

7. Remain centered on current concern. ____ ____ ____ _____

8. Assist client in clarifying experience. ____ ____ ____ _____

9. Communicate understanding. ____ ____ ____ _____

10. Use open questions to explore alternatives. ____ ____ ____ _____

11. Offer reassurance. ____ ____ ____ _____

12. Explore available support services, and refer as appropriate. ____ ____ ____ _____

13. Use Completion Protocol. ____ ____ ____ _____

Evaluation

1. Ask client for feedback on effectiveness of support or comfort provided. ____ ____ ____ _____

2. Observe verbal and nonverbal responses. ____ ____ ____ _____

3. Identify support systems available. ____ ____ ____ _____

• Identify unexpected outcomes and intervene as necessary. ____ ____ ____ _____

• Record and report intervention and client's response. ____ ____ ____ _____

Performance Checklist: Skill 2.3

Active Listening

	S	U	NP	Comments

Assessment

1. Assess client's pattern of communication with caregivers. ____ ____ ____ _____

2. Identify sensory or neurological alterations. ____ ____ ____ _____

3. Identify cultural influences. ____ ____ ____ _____

Implementation

1. Use Standard Protocol. ____ ____ ____ _____

2. Use nonverbal communication to convey interest. ____ ____ ____ _____
   a. Sit within 4 feet of client, maintaining good eye contact. ____ ____ ____ _____
   b. Maintain open, relaxed posture. ____ ____ ____ _____

3. Use open-ended questions in logical sequence. ____ ____ ____ _____

4. Listen attentively without interrupting. ____ ____ ____ _____

5. Give feedback or paraphrase as appropriate. ____ ____ ____ _____

6. Clarify unclear messages. ____ ____ ____ _____

7. Focus on main concerns. ____ ____ ____ _____

8. Identify incongruencies. ____ ____ ____ _____

9. Allow silence. ____ ____ ____ _____

10. Summarize observations to client. ____ ____ ____ _____

11. Use Completion Protocol. ____ ____ ____ _____

Evaluation

1. Identify factors that facilitate or interfere with communication. ____ ____ ____ _____

2. Determine accuracy of interpretation of communication. ____ ____ ____ _____

• Identify unexpected outcomes and intervene as necessary. ____ ____ ____ _____

• Record and report intervention and client's response. ____ ____ ____ _____

Performance Checklist: Skill 2.4

Interviewing

	S	U	NP	Comments

Assessment

1. Review available client information.

2. Identify psychological or physiological factors that may interfere with process (pain or anxiety).

3. Assess client's current sensory or neurological status.

Implementation

1. Use Standard Protocol.

2. Orientation phase
   a. Greet client and significant others.
   b. Provide privacy.
   c. Sit facing client.
   d. Determine whether client is able to proceed.

3. Working phase
   a. Keep on focus.
   b. Seek chronological account.
   c. Observe nonverbal cues.
   d. For each symptom, determine onset, precipitating factors, quality of characteristics, region, severity, and timing.
   e. Clarify absence of other symptoms.
   f. Identify past hospitalizations.
   g. Identify OTC medications used regularly.
   h. Identify other prescribed medications used.
   i. Identify risk factors.
   j. Continue with other areas of interest or concern.

4. Termination phase (prepare client for closing, summarize)
   a. Provide client with idea that interview is nearly finished.
   b. Summarize your understanding of client's health concerns.

5. Use Completion Protocol.

	S	U	NP	Comments

Evaluation

1. Ask client if adequate opportunity was provided to describe concerns.

    ____ ____ ____ _____

2. Determine congruence of verbal and nonverbal communication.

    ____ ____ ____ _____

• Identify unexpected outcomes and intervene as necessary.

    ____ ____ ____ _____

• Record and report intervention and client's response.

    ____ ____ ____ _____

Name _____ Date _____ Instructor's Name _____

Performance Checklist: Skill 2.5

Communicating with an Anxious Client

	S	U	NP	Comments

Assessment

1. Assess for physical, behavioral, and verbal cues indicating anxiety.

2. Assess for possible factors causing client anxiety.

3. Assess factors influencing communication with client.

4. Assess own level of anxiety, making conscious effort to remain calm.

Implementation

1. Use Standard Protocol.

2. Provide brief, simple introduction of self and role.

3. Use appropriate nonverbal behaviors and active listening skills.

4. Use clear and concise verbal techniques.

5. Assist client to acquire alternate coping strategies.

6. Minimize noise in physical setting.

7. Adjust amount of time for communication depending on client's needs.

8. Use Completion Protocol.

Evaluation

1. Have client discuss ways to cope with anxiety in the future.

2. Observe level of anxiety.

3. Evaluate client's ability to discuss factors causing anxiety.

• Identify unexpected outcomes and intervene as necessary.

• Record and report intervention and client's response.

Name _____ Date _____ Instructor's Name _____

Performance Checklist: Skill 2.6

Verbally Deescalating a Potentially Violent Client

	S	U	NP	Comments

Assessment

1. Observe for behaviors or expressions that indicate client anger. ____ ____ ____ _____

2. Assess factors that influence communication of angry client. ____ ____ ____ _____

3. Consider available resources to assist in communication with angry client. ____ ____ ____ _____

Implementation

1. Use Standard Protocol. ____ ____ ____ _____

2. Create a climate of acceptance for client with nonthreatening communication skills. ____ ____ ____ _____

3. Respond appropriately to client by using therapeutic silence, allowing client to ventilate feelings. ____ ____ ____ _____

4. Set limits on power-struggle questions. Remain calm without arguing. ____ ____ ____ _____

5. Encourage client to write about negative thoughts. ____ ____ ____ _____

6. Encourage physical exercise to redirect energy. ____ ____ ____ _____

7. Remain calm and continue to set limits on inappropriate behavior. ____ ____ ____ _____

8. Maintain own personal space and safety. Maintain nonthreatening body language. ____ ____ ____ _____

Nurse Alert: Avoid touch.

9. Adjust amount and quality of time depending on client's needs. ____ ____ ____ _____

10. Explore alternatives in order to prevent future episodes of anger. ____ ____ ____ _____

11. Use Completion Protocol. ____ ____ ____ _____

	S	U	NP	Comments

Evaluation

1. Ask if feelings of anger have subsided.   ___ ___ ___ _____

2. Determine client's ability to answer questions.   ___ ___ ___ _____

• Identify unexpected outcomes and intervene as necessary.   ___ ___ ___ _____

• Record and report intervention and client's response.   ___ ___ ___ _____

Performance Checklist: Skill 3.1

Handwashing and Disinfection

	S	U	NP	Comments

Assessment

1. Assess client's risk for, or extent of, infection. ___ ___ ___ _____
2. Inspect integrity of your hands and nails. ___ ___ ___ _____
3. Keep natural nails less than ¼ inch long. ___ ___ ___ _____
4. Consider the type of nursing activity being performed. ___ ___ ___ _____
5. Inspect hands for visible soiling. ___ ___ ___ _____

Implementation

1. Remove wristwatch and rings. ___ ___ ___ _____
2. Keep hands and uniform away from sink surfaces. ___ ___ ___ _____
3. Turn on water. ___ ___ ___ _____
4. Avoid splashing. ___ ___ ___ _____
5. Regulate flow and water temperature. ___ ___ ___ _____
6. Wet hands, keeping hands lower than elbows. ___ ___ ___ _____
7. Apply 3 to 5 ml soap and lather thoroughly. ___ ___ ___ _____
8. Interlace fingers and rub palms and back of hands with a circular motion at least five times each, keeping fingertips pointed down. ___ ___ ___ _____
9. Clean under fingernails. ___ ___ ___ _____

Nurse Alert: Do not tear or cut skin under or around nail.

10. Rinse thoroughly, keeping hands lower than elbows. ___ ___ ___ _____
11. Repeat steps 1 through 9 if hands are heavily soiled. ___ ___ ___ _____
12. Dry hands thoroughly from fingers to wrists to forearms. ___ ___ ___ _____
13. Discard paper towel, if used. ___ ___ ___ _____
14. Turn off water, using dry paper towel or foot or knee pedals. ___ ___ ___ _____
15. Use individual-use container of lotion or barrier cream if hands are dry or chapped. ___ ___ ___ _____

	S	U	NP	Comments

16. Antiseptic handrub
   a. Apply adequate amount of product to cover hands and fingers. _____ _____ _____ _____
   b. Rub hands together, covering all surfaces, until hands are dry. _____ _____ _____ _____

Evaluation

1. Inspect surfaces of hands for obvious soil. _____ _____ _____ _____

2. Inspect for dermatitis or cracking. _____ _____ _____ _____

Performance Checklist: Skill 3.2

Using Disposable Clean Gloves

	S	U	NP	Comments
1. Application				
a. Inspect for cuts, abrasions, or wounds that indicate need for gloves.	___	___	___	_____
b. Inspect skin for redness, inflammation, dryness, or vesicles indicating latex allergy.	___	___	___	_____
c. Select appropriate type and size of gloves. Put on gloves (no special technique) to cover wrists.	___	___	___	_____
d. Interlink fingers to ensure a proper, comfortable fit.	___	___	___	_____
2. Removal				
a. Remove first glove, touching only glove to glove.	___	___	___	_____
b. Pull glove inside out and discard.	___	___	___	_____
c. Remove second glove, touching only inside of glove, turning inside out and discard.	___	___	___	_____
3. Evaluation				
a. Perform hand hygiene.	___	___	___	_____

Performance Checklist: Skill 3.3

Caring for Clients Under Isolation Precautions

	S	U	NP	Comments

Assessment

1. Review agency protocol and precautions for specific isolation systems and the reason for isolation.

    _____ _____ _____ _____

2. Review appropriate laboratory results.

    _____ _____ _____ _____

3. Consider type of care to be provided while in client's room; gather all necessary equipment before entering.

    _____ _____ _____ _____

4. Assess client's and family's understanding of isolation precautions.

    _____ _____ _____ _____

5. Identify if client has a known latex allergy.

    _____ _____ _____ _____

Implementation

1. Use Standard Protocol.

    _____ _____ _____ _____

2. Enter client's room and remain by the door. Introduce yourself and purpose of visit.

    _____ _____ _____ _____

3. Prepare for entering the room.
    a. Apply mask.
    b. Apply eyewear or goggles, as appropriate.
    c. Apply gown.
    d. Apply disposable gloves.

    _____ _____ _____ _____
    _____ _____ _____ _____
    _____ _____ _____ _____
    _____ _____ _____ _____

4. Enter client's room and arrange supplies and equipment.

    _____ _____ _____ _____

5. Assess vital signs.

    _____ _____ _____ _____

Nurse Alert: Dispose of sharps in puncture-resistant container. Equipment remains in room if vancomycin-resistant enterococcus (VCE) is present.

6. Administer medications.

    _____ _____ _____ _____

Nurse Alert: Hepatitis B and C are spread through parenteral or percutaneous exposure to tainted blood.

7. Administer hygienic care.

    _____ _____ _____ _____

8. Collect specimens.

    _____ _____ _____ _____

9. Dispose of linens and trash.

    _____ _____ _____ _____

	S	U	NP	Comments

10. Remove all reusable equipment, as appropriate. Clean contaminated surfaces. ___ ___ ___ _____

11. Resupply room. ___ ___ ___ _____

12. Leave isolation room. Remove barriers.
   a. Remove gloves, touching only outside, and discard. ___ ___ ___ _____
   b. Remove mask, touching only ties. ___ ___ ___ _____
   c. Untie neck of gown, then back strings. Remove hands from sleeves without touching outside of gown. ___ ___ ___ _____
   d. Fold gown inside out and place in laundry bag or garbage (disposable gown). ___ ___ ___ _____
   e. Remove goggles without touching hair or face. ___ ___ ___ _____
   f. Wash hands. ___ ___ ___ _____
   g. Retrieve watch and stethoscope. ___ ___ ___ _____
   h. Leave room and close door. ___ ___ ___ _____

13. Use Completion Protocol. ___ ___ ___ _____

Evaluation

1. Evaluate client's and family's understanding of precautions. ___ ___ ___ _____

2. Monitor clinical status of neighboring clients. ___ ___ ___ _____

• Identify unexpected outcomes and intervene as necessary. ___ ___ ___ _____

• Record and report intervention and client's response. ___ ___ ___ _____

Performance Checklist: Skill 3.4

Special Tuberculosis Precautions

	S	U	NP	Comments

Assessment

1. Assess client's current health status and potential for tuberculosis. _____ _____ _____ _____

2. Consult with engineering department to assess effectiveness of negative airflow using flutter strip or smoke stick. _____ _____ _____ _____

3. Consider type of care measures to be performed. _____ _____ _____ _____

Implementation

1. Use Standard Protocol. _____ _____ _____ _____

2. Apply recommended mask before entering room. _____ _____ _____ _____

3. Explain purpose of AFB isolation to client and family (droplets suspended in air). _____ _____ _____ _____

4. Instruct client to cover mouth with tissue when coughing and to wear mask when leaving room. _____ _____ _____ _____

Nurse Alert: Particulate respiratory mask is not to be placed on client.

5. Provide client care. _____ _____ _____ _____

6. Leave room and close the door. _____ _____ _____ _____

7. Remove respiratory protective device. _____ _____ _____ _____

8. Check agency policy for number of uses for protective devices before disposal. _____ _____ _____ _____

9. Use Completion Protocol. _____ _____ _____ _____

Evaluation

1. Assess labs for repeat AFB smears. _____ _____ _____ _____

2. Evaluate client's and family's understanding of how tuberculosis is transmitted. _____ _____ _____ _____

3. Check for suspected respiratory symptoms in neighboring clients. _____ _____ _____ _____

• Identify unexpected outcomes and intervene as necessary. _____ _____ _____ _____

• Record and report intervention and client's response. _____ _____ _____ _____

Performance Checklist: Skill 4.1

Creating and Maintaining a Sterile Field

	S	U	NP	Comments

Assessment

1. Verify that procedure requires surgical aseptic technique.

2. Assess client's comfort needs before procedure.

3. Assess for latex allergies.

4. Check commercially prepared sterile kits for integrity and expiration date.

5. Anticipate number and variety of supplies needed.

Implementation

1. Use Standard Protocol.

2. Apply cap, mask, protective eyewear, and gown.

3. Prepare clean, dry work surface at or above waist level.

4. Open *commercially* prepared or agency processed kit without contaminating contents.
   a. Place kit or package on work surface.
   b. Remove outer wrap and discard.
   c. Grasp outer surface of tip of outermost flap.
   d. Open first flap away from yourself.
   e. Open left or right side flap without reaching over sterile field.
   f. Open other side flap.
   g. Pull last flap toward yourself.

5. Prepare a paper supply bundle.
   a. Place package on work surface. Remove outer wrap, if present. Remove indicator tape and discard.
   b. Open outer layer as in step 4 c–g. Use opened paper wrapper as sterile field.

	S	U	NP	Comments

6. Prepare sterile drape.
   a. Place pack on work surface.
   b. Grasp folded edge of drape and lift from wrapper.
   c. Allow drape to unfold, keeping it above waist level.
   d. Grasp adjacent corner of drape and hold straight over work surface.
   e. Position drape over top half then bottom half of work surface.

7. Add packaged items to sterile field.
   a. Open sterile item by peeling back outer wrapper.
   b. Place onto field at an angle so that arm does not reach over field.
   c. Dispose of outer wrapper.

8. Pour sterile solutions without splashing.
   a. Verify type of solution and expiration date.
   b. Remove cap and sterile seal, keeping inside of cap sterile.
   c. Slowly pour from a safe distance without splashing.
   d. Pour a small amount into nonsterile receptacle, if solution container was previously opened.
   e. Label container with date and time (consider contaminated after 24 hours).

9. Proceed with sterile procedure.

Evaluation

1. Evaluate client for signs of infection in 48 hours.

2. Inspect for redness, edema, warmth, odor, and drainage.

• Identify unexpected outcomes and intervene as necessary.

• Record and report intervention and client's response.

Performance Checklist: Skill 4.2

Sterile Gloving

	S	U	NP	Comments

Assessment

1. Verify that procedure requires sterile gloves. ____ ____ ____ _____

2. Check for latex allergy/sensitivity. ____ ____ ____ _____

3. Inspect condition of hands. ____ ____ ____ _____

Implementation

1. Use Standard Protocol. ____ ____ ____ _____

2. Check integrity of glove package. ____ ____ ____ _____

3. Remove outer package wrapper using sterile technique. ____ ____ ____ _____

4. Open inner wrapper. ____ ____ ____ _____

5. Identify right and left gloves. ____ ____ ____ _____

6. Glove dominant hand first, touching only inside of glove. ____ ____ ____ _____

7. With gloved hand, slide fingers under cuff of glove for nondominant hand. Pull glove onto nondominant hand without touching exposed skin, keeping thumb of dominant hand abducted back. ____ ____ ____ _____

8. Interlock fingers of gloved hands, holding hands away from body. ____ ____ ____ _____

9. Proceed with intended procedure. ____ ____ ____ _____

Glove Removal

10. Grasp outside of one cuff with gloved hand and pull off, turning glove inside out. Discard glove. ____ ____ ____ _____

11. Remove remaining glove by placing fingers of bare hand under cuff and pull off, turning glove inside out. Discard glove. ____ ____ ____ _____

12. Use Completion Protocol. ____ ____ ____ _____

	S	U	NP	Comments

Evaluation

1. Assess for signs of infection within 48 hours.

   ___ ___ ___ _____

2. Inspect treated area for localized signs of infection.

   ___ ___ ___ _____

- Identify unexpected outcomes and intervene as necessary.

   ___ ___ ___ _____

- Record and report intervention and client's response.

   ___ ___ ___ _____

Performance Checklist: Skill 5.1

Safety Equipment and Fall Prevention

	S	U	NP	Comments

Assessment

1. Assess client's age, level of consciousness, degree of orientation, ability to follow directions, and ability to cooperate. ____ ____ ____ _____

2. Assess client's medical history and medications. ____ ____ ____ _____

3. Assess the environment for potential safety hazards. ____ ____ ____ _____

4. Assess degree of assistance needed by client. ____ ____ ____ _____

Implementation

1. Use Standard Protocol. ____ ____ ____ _____

Nurse Alert: Before using any equipment, be sure you know safety features and proper use.

2. Explain use of call bell or intercom.
   a. Provide client with glasses and/or hearing aid, if used. ____ ____ ____ _____
   b. Demonstrate use of call bell or intercom to client/family. ____ ____ ____ _____
   c. Have client and family return— demonstrate use. ____ ____ ____ _____
   d. Explain when call bell is to be used. ____ ____ ____ _____
   e. Secure call bell in accessible location. ____ ____ ____ _____

3. Describe use of hospital bed and side rails.
   a. Keep bed in low position with wheels locked. ____ ____ ____ _____
   b. Explain purpose of side rails to client and family. ____ ____ ____ _____
   c. Check agency policy regarding side rail use. ____ ____ ____ _____
   d. Keep side rails up for clients at risk for falls. ____ ____ ____ _____
   e. Leave one side rail down for ambulatory clients. ____ ____ ____ _____

4. Arrange necessary items within client's reach. ____ ____ ____ _____

5. Provide adequate, nonglare lighting. ____ ____ ____ _____

6. Remove unnecessary objects from area. ____ ____ ____ _____

	S	U	NP	Comments

7. Provide safe transport using a wheelchair.
   a. Lock both wheels for client transfers.   _____ _____ _____ _____
   b. Raise footplates before transfer. Lower footplates and place client's feet on them after transfer.   _____ _____ _____ _____
   c. Have client sit well back in seat with seat belt on.   _____ _____ _____ _____
   d. Back wheelchair into and out of elevators.   _____ _____ _____ _____
   e. Back down ramps or inclines.   _____ _____ _____ _____

8. Provide safe transport using a stretcher.
   a. Lock wheels during transfers.   _____ _____ _____ _____
   b. Use safety belts across client's upper thighs or raise rails.   _____ _____ _____ _____
   c. Push stretcher from the end where client's head rests.   _____ _____ _____ _____
   d. Enter elevator head first.   _____ _____ _____ _____

Nurse Alert: Clients should not be left on stretchers unattended.

9. Assisting the client with ambulation:
   a. Explain safety measures.   _____ _____ _____ _____
   b. Have client take a few steps while standing by the stronger side.   _____ _____ _____ _____
   c. Support client with arm closest to client on gait belt or around waist.   _____ _____ _____ _____
   d. Take a few steps forward with client, assessing strength and balance.   _____ _____ _____ _____
   e. Return client to bed or chair if weak or dizzy.   _____ _____ _____ _____

10. Use Completion Protocol.   _____ _____ _____ _____

Evaluation

1. Identify client's response to safety measures.   _____ _____ _____ _____

2. Observe appropriate use of call bell.   _____ _____ _____ _____

3. Evaluate client's and family's use of the equipment.   _____ _____ _____ _____

• Identify unexpected outcomes and intervene as necessary.   _____ _____ _____ _____

• Record and report intervention and client's response.   _____ _____ _____ _____

Performance Checklist: Skill 5.2

Designing a Restraint-Free Environment

	S	U	NP	Comments

Assessment

1. Identify factors that place the client at risk for injury.

2. Review medications taken by client that increase risk for falls.

3. Assess client's orientation to time, place, and person.

4. Observe client's behavior to document specific risks for injury.

Implementation

1. Use Standard Protocol.

2. Orient client and family to surroundings.

3. Encourage family and friends to stay with client.

4. Place client in a room close to nurse's station.

5. Provide visual and auditory stimuli (clock, radio, calendar).

6. Encourage family and friends to provide personal items of client's.

7. Provide same caregivers whenever possible.

8. Respond promptly to client's needs and requests.

Nurse Alert: Getting out of bed for toileting purposes is a common event that leads to falls.

9. Organize a predictable daily routine.

10. Use wedge pillows in chair with thick part in front.

11. Use pressure-sensitive monitoring device.
    a. Explain and demonstrate use of device to family and friends.
    b. Measure the client's thigh circumference.
    c. Test battery and alarm.
    d. Apply leg band just above the knee and secure in place.

	S	U	NP	Comments

    e. Explain when alarm will sound.

    f. Deactivate device when assisting client to ambulate.

12. Use stress-reduction techniques for client (i.e., massage, guided imagery).

13. Use music, audio books, and videos selected specifically for client.

14. Position catheters, tubes, and drains out of client's view.

15. Consult with physical therapist, speech therapist, and occupational therapist for activities to provide stimulation.

16. Use Completion Protocol.

Evaluation

1. Review incidence of behaviors that increase risk of injury for self or others.

2. Verify absence of violence toward others.

- Identify unexpected outcomes and intervene as necessary.

- Record and report intervention and client's response.

Performance Checklist: Skill 5.3

Applying Physical Restraints

	S	U	NP	Comments

Assessment

1. Assess need for restraints when all other measures have failed.

2. Review agency policy regarding restraints.

3. Review manufacturer's instructions for application.

4. Inspect area where restraint is to be placed, including skin integrity and circulation, presence of IVs and AV shunt.

Nurse Alert: Select the least restrictive type of restraint. Avoid interferences with therapeutic equipment.

Implementation

1. Use Standard Protocol.

2. Place client in proper body alignment.

3. Pad bony prominences where restraints will be placed.

4. Apply properly sized restraints.
   a. Jacket restraint
   b. Belt restraint (avoid restricting ventilation)
   c. Extremity, or limb, restraint (used in lateral position)
   d. Mitten restraint

5. Attach restraints to bed frame.

Nurse Alert: Do not attach to side rails.

6. Apply jacket restraint for client in a chair with ties under armrests and secured at back.

7. Use quick-release ties.

8. Attend to client's needs before leaving, identifying when you will return. Make sure call bell is within reach.

Nurse Alert: Responding and providing for client's ADLs is essential.

9. Check restraints every 60 minutes for placement, and circulation and mobility to the area.

	S	U	NP	Comments

10. Release restraints q2h and complete range of motion to site.   _____ _____ _____ _____

11. Use Completion Protocol.   _____ _____ _____ _____

Evaluation

1. Evaluate effectiveness of restraint used.   _____ _____ _____ _____

2. Verify prescribed therapies are continued without interruption.   _____ _____ _____ _____

3. Reassess client's need for restraint at least every 24 hours.   _____ _____ _____ _____

- Identify unexpected outcomes and intervene as necessary.   _____ _____ _____ _____

- Record and report intervention and client's response.   _____ _____ _____ _____

Performance Checklist: Skill 5.4

Seizure Precautions

	S	U	NP	Comments

Assessment

1. Assess client's type and frequency of seizures.

2. Assess for factors that may precipitate a client's seizures.

3. Inspect the client's environment for potential safety hazards.

Implementation

1. Use Standard Protocol.

2. Prepare bed with padded side rails and headboard and bed in lowest position.

3. Provide or encourage use of a bracelet or ID card noting seizure disorder.

4. If a seizure occurs:
   a. Stay with the client. Protect head from injury.
   b. Provide privacy, if possible.
   c. Observe sequence and timing of seizure activity, along with client's color and respirations.
   d. Insert oral airway if needed for client with status epilepticus.
   e. Assess client after seizure.
   f. Explain to client what happened and provide a quiet environment.

Nurse Alert: Do not place objects or fingers near client's mouth.

Evaluation

1. Assess for injury during and after the seizure.

2. Observe respiratory status during and after the seizure.

3. Ask client to verbalize feelings.

4. Provide privacy, quiet, and nonstimulating environment.

	S	U	NP	Comments

- Identify unexpected outcomes and intervene as necessary. ___ ___ ___ _____

- Record and report intervention and client's response. ___ ___ ___ _____

Performance Checklist: Skill 5.5

Safety Measures for Radioactive Materials

	S	U	NP	Comments

Assessment

1. Consult with radiation safety officer to identify type and amount of radiation to be used, its side effects, and hazards. _____ _____ _____ _____

2. Identify restrictions related to time and distance. _____ _____ _____ _____

Nurse Alert: Keep time of exposure to caregivers within a safe limit.

Implementation

1. Use Standard Protocol. _____ _____ _____ _____

2. Explain treatment plan to client and family. _____ _____ _____ _____

3. Prepare a private room, posting use of radiation on door and marking safe distances on floor. _____ _____ _____ _____

4. Provide client with diversional activities. _____ _____ _____ _____

5. Explain safety regulations to client and visitors. _____ _____ _____ _____

6. Keep track of exposure time using badge. _____ _____ _____ _____

7. Wear shields when providing care. Wash gloves before removal and dispose of appropriately. Wash hands thoroughly. _____ _____ _____ _____

8. Identify special requirements for laboratory specimens, dietary trays, drainage and secretions, linens, and trash. _____ _____ _____ _____

9. Request discharge survey to ensure that all sources of radiation were removed after treatment. _____ _____ _____ _____

10. Use Completion Protocol. _____ _____ _____ _____

Evaluation

1. Evaluate amount of radiation exposure of client, visitors, and staff. _____ _____ _____ _____

• Identify unexpected outcomes and intervene as necessary. _____ _____ _____ _____

• Record and report intervention and client's response. _____ _____ _____ _____

Performance Checklist: Skill 6.1

Assisting with Moving and Positioning Clients in Bed

	S	U	NP	Comments

Assessment

1. Assess client's age, weight, level of consciousness, and ability and willingness to participate. _____ _____ _____ _____

2. Assess muscle strength and joint mobility. _____ _____ _____ _____

3. Assess need for analgesic 30 to 60 minutes before position changes. _____ _____ _____ _____
4. Assess for therapeutic equipment. _____ _____ _____ _____

Implementation

1. Use Standard Protocol. _____ _____ _____ _____

2. Raise level of bed to comfortable working height. _____ _____ _____ _____

3. Remove all pillows and devices. _____ _____ _____ _____

4. Get extra help, as needed. _____ _____ _____ _____

5. Position client:
   a. Moving dependent client up in bed with one nurse and client assistance:
      (1) Adjust position of equipment (e.g., IV line). _____ _____ _____ _____
      (2) Provide client with glasses or hearing aid, if needed. _____ _____ _____ _____
      (3) Lower head of bed, lower side rail nearest you, and remove pillow. _____ _____ _____ _____
      (4) Assist client to flex knees and place feet flat. _____ _____ _____ _____
      (5) Support client under shoulders and upper back. _____ _____ _____ _____
      (6) If trapeze is available, assist client to grasp it and support client under lower body. _____ _____ _____ _____
      (7) Have client lift and push with feet on a count of three. Repeat as necessary. _____ _____ _____ _____
      (8) Ask client about level of comfort. _____ _____ _____ _____

Nurse Alert: Use principles of body mechanics.

   b. Assisting client to move up in bed when client cannot assist: _____ _____ _____ _____

	S	U	NP	Comments

(1) Remove pillow and lower head of bed. ____ ____ ____ _____

(2) Roll client onto pull sheet. ____ ____ ____ _____

(3) Grasp pull sheet firmly with both hands. ____ ____ ____ _____

(4) Face head of bed with feet apart for support. ____ ____ ____ _____

(5) Ask client to lift head and place arms across body. ____ ____ ____ _____

(6) Move client (on a count of three) toward head of bed. ____ ____ ____ _____

(7) Position client comfortably. ____ ____ ____ _____

c. Positioning client in semi-Fowler's and Fowler's position:

(1) Raise head of bed to correct level. ____ ____ ____ _____

(2) Use pillows to support client's arms and hands. ____ ____ ____ _____

(3) Position pillow under client's head and raise knee break slightly, avoiding pressure on popliteal space. ____ ____ ____ _____

(4) Change degree of elevation frequently. ____ ____ ____ _____

(5) Identify five pressure points. ____ ____ ____ _____

d. Moving dependent client to lateral position:

(1) Lower the head of the bed. ____ ____ ____ _____

(2) Move client to side of bed opposite where client will be turned. ____ ____ ____ _____

(3) From other side of bed, assist client to raise arm nearest you above head. ____ ____ ____ _____

(4) Grasp client's shoulder and hip and assist client to roll toward you. ____ ____ ____ _____

(5) Flex client's upper leg and support from knee to foot. ____ ____ ____ _____

(6) Ease client's shoulder forward. ____ ____ ____ _____

(7) Support upper arm level with shoulder. ____ ____ ____ _____

(8) Support client's back. ____ ____ ____ _____

(9) Make sure that client is in alignment. ____ ____ ____ _____

(10) Identify pressure points. ____ ____ ____ _____

e. Log-rolling client to maintain neck and spinal alignment:

(1) Determine number of staff required to assist. ____ ____ ____ _____

(2) Lower the head of the bed. ____ ____ ____ _____

(3) Place a pillow between client's legs. Position pull sheet between shoulders and knees. ____ ____ ____ _____

(4) Cross client's arms on chest. ____ ____ ____ _____

(5) With two caregivers on same side, support upper and lower body. Another cargiver is on the other side of the bed. ____ ____ ____ _____

(6) On a count of three, turn client in one continual, smooth movement. ____ ____ ____ _____

	S	U	NP	Comments

(7) Place pillow supports as with the side-lying position.   _____ _____ _____ _____

  f. Moving dependent client to Sims' (semiprone) position: _____ _____ _____ _____

    (1) In lateral position, externally rotate arm against mattress and extend lowermost leg.   _____ _____ _____ _____

    (2) Support client's upper arm and leg in flexed positions.   _____ _____ _____ _____

    (3) Identify eight pressure points.   _____ _____ _____ _____

  g. Positioning dependent client in supine position:

    (1) Place client on back with head flat.   _____ _____ _____ _____

    (2) Place pillow under upper shoulders, neck, and head.   _____ _____ _____ _____

    (3) Place trochanter rolls at hips.   _____ _____ _____ _____

    (4) Place small supports under ankles. Footboard may be used.   _____ _____ _____ _____

    (5) Place small supports under forearms and rolls in hands.   _____ _____ _____ _____

    (6) Identify pressure points.   _____ _____ _____ _____

  h. Positioning client in prone position:

    (1) Roll client to one side.   _____ _____ _____ _____

    (2) Roll client over, keeping elbow straight and hand under hip.   _____ _____ _____ _____

    (3) Turn client's head to the side and support with small pillow.   _____ _____ _____ _____

    (4) Place a small pillow under client's abdomen below diaphragm.   _____ _____ _____ _____

    (5) Support arms in flexed position level with shoulders.   _____ _____ _____ _____

    (6) Support lower legs with pillow to elevate toes.   _____ _____ _____ _____

6. Use Completion Protocol.   _____ _____ _____ _____

Evaluation

1. Inspect skin for pressure areas (reactive hyperemia). Observe again after 60 minutes.   _____ _____ _____ _____

2. Ask if client is comfortable.   _____ _____ _____ _____

3. Observe body alignment and positioning.   _____ _____ _____ _____

4. Ask client to state benefits of positioning.   _____ _____ _____ _____

• Identify unexpected outcomes and intervene as necessary.   _____ _____ _____ _____

• Record and report intervention and client's response.   _____ _____ _____ _____

Performance Checklist: Skill 6.2

Minimizing Orthostatic Hypotension

	S	U	NP	Comments

Assessment

1. Check prior blood pressure and pulse readings and client's activity level. ____ ____ ____ _____

2. Assess factors that may precipitate hypotension. ____ ____ ____ _____

Implementation

1. Use Standard Protocol. ____ ____ ____ _____

2. Explain reason for gradual position change. ____ ____ ____ _____

3. Raise head of bed slowly to determine client's tolerance. Instruct client to report dizziness or lightheadedness. ____ ____ ____ _____

4. Allow client to dangle legs if appropriate. Encourage client to move shoulders in circles and flex and extend ankles and knees. Reassess blood pressure. ____ ____ ____ _____

5. Proceed with planned activity. ____ ____ ____ _____

Nurse Alert: Do not attempt to ambulate if client reports dizziness, nausea, or appears pale.

6. Use Completion Protocol. ____ ____ ____ _____

Evaluation

1. Continue to observe client for signs of weakness or dizziness. ____ ____ ____ _____

2. Obtain blood pressure, pulse, and respirations if client experiences weakness or dizziness. ____ ____ ____ _____

3. Ask client to describe interventions to minimize hypotension and prevent injury. ____ ____ ____ _____

• Identify unexpected outcomes and intervene as necessary. ____ ____ ____ _____

• Record and report intervention and client's response. ____ ____ ____ _____

Performance Checklist: Skill 6.3

Transferring from Bed to Chair

	S	U	NP	Comments

Assessment

1. Assess muscle strength of extremities.

2. Assess joint mobility and history of osteoporosis.

3. Assess vision, hearing, sensation, and altered sensation.

4. Assess ability and motivation to participate.

5. Determine presence and location of equipment and tubing (e.g., IV, Foley catheter, drains).

6. Assess need for analgesic medication before transfer.

Implementation

1. Use Standard Protocol.

2. Position chair or wheelchair so that move will be toward client's stronger side.

3. Lower bed to lowest position. Lower side rail. Turn client to one side with the knees flexed.

Nurse Alert: Obtain assistance, if necessary, for safe transfer of client.

4. Raise head of bed to highest level.

5. Face client with your feet apart.

6. Assist client to sitting position by lifting upper body and swinging client's legs over edge of bed.

7. Encourage client to assist as much as possible.

8. Instruct client to take deep breath and to sit for 1 to 2 minutes.

9. Assist client to put on nonskid slippers or shoes.

10. Spread feet apart. Flex and align hips and knees.

	S	U	NP	Comments

11. Apply gait belt if needed for support. Apply sling if needed for flaccid arm.

Nurse Alert: A gait or walking belt should be used in place of the under axilla technique.

12. Grasp transfer belt, keeping back straight and wide base of support. Have client place hands on your shoulder (not around neck).

13. Rock client forward to a standing position on a count of three.

14. Keep foot against client's foot and knee against client's knee for support.

15. Pivot client toward seat of chair, with client reaching for chair arm.

16. Assist client to ease into chair, and attain proper alignment.

17. Flex hips and knees while lowering client into chair.

18. Observe client for proper alignment. Provide pillows for support.

19. Use Completion Protocol.

Evaluation

1. Evaluate client's ability to participate in the transfer.

2. Monitor length of time in chair and ability to shift weight.

3. Observe response to position changes.

• Identify unexpected outcomes and intervene as necessary.

• Record and report intervention and client's response.

Performance Checklist: Skill 6.4

Using a Mechanical (Hoyer) Lift for Transfer from Bed to Chair

	S	U	NP	Comments

Assessment

1. Compare weight limit for lift with client's current weight.

2. Assess muscle strength and mobility of extremities.

3. Assess vital signs.

4. Assess client's level of motivation.

Implementation

1. Use Standard Protocol.

2. Obtain additional caregiver for assistance. Move lift to bedside and place a comfortable chair in a convenient location.

3. Raise bed to working height. Turn client to the side and place canvas sling from head to knees.

4. Instruct client to keep arms crossed over body. Position lift with base spread and under bed.

5. Attach lift chains to sling. Adjust sling to evenly distribute client's weight.

6. Raise lift slightly.

7. Adjust sling as necessary.

8. Pump the lift and guide client's legs over side of bed. Protect client's head and extremities from injury.

9. Instruct client to keep arms folded.

10. Check position of chair and guide lift over so that client will be positioned appropriately.

Nurse Alert: Stabilize chair, wheelchair, or commode.

11. Release lift value slowly, lower client into chair, and release lift chains.

	S	U	NP	Comments

12. Use Completion Protocol. ___ ___ ___ _____

Evaluation

1. Ask client's response to transfer. ___ ___ ___ _____

2. Evaluate client's ability to tolerate the transfer and being out of bed in the chair. ___ ___ ___ _____

3. Observe body alignment. ___ ___ ___ _____

4. Compare vital signs with baseline. ___ ___ ___ _____

• Identify unexpected outcomes and intervene as necessary. ___ ___ ___ _____

• Record and report intervention and client's response. ___ ___ ___ _____

Performance Checklist: Skill 6.5

Transferring from Bed to Stretcher

| | S | U | NP | Comments |

Assessment

1. Assess client's level of consciousness and ability to participate in the transfer. ____ ____ ____ _____

2. Assess joint mobility and limitations. ____ ____ ____ _____

3. Assess presence of pain and offer analgesic if needed. ____ ____ ____ _____

Implementation

1. Use Standard Protocol. ____ ____ ____ _____

2. Position bed flat. Raise bed to same height as stretcher. Lower side rails. ____ ____ ____ _____

3. Cover client with sheet or bath blanket. Remove topmost covers. ____ ____ ____ _____

4. Check for position of equipment or tubes (e.g., IV, Foley). ____ ____ ____ _____

5. Position stretcher as close as possible to bed, with wheels locked and side rails down. ____ ____ ____ _____

6. To transfer with client assistance:
   a. Stand near side of stretcher and instruct client to move feet, buttocks, then upper body over to stretcher.
   b. Check that client is in center of stretcher. ____ ____ ____ _____

7. To transfer without client assistance:
   a. Place pull sheet so that it supports from client's head to midthighs.
   b. Roll pull sheet close to client's body. Assist client to cross arms over chest. ____ ____ ____ _____
   c. Two caregivers are positioned on one side of bed, two caregivers on side of stretcher, and one caregiver stands at foot of bed to move client's feet.
   d. Lift on a count of three and move client over to edge of bed. ____ ____ ____ _____
   e. With another coordinated lift, move client to stretcher. ____ ____ ____ _____

Nurse Alert: As many as five caregivers may be required for a heavy client who cannot assist.

	S	U	NP	Comments

8. Raise both side rails and head of stretcher, if not contraindicated.

9. Instruct client to keep hands inside and off side rails of stretcher while it is moving.

10. Use Completion Protocol.

Evaluation

1. Evaluate client's ability to participate in and tolerate the transfer.

2. Ask how the transfer felt.

3. Ask response to change in environment.

•   Identify unexpected outcomes and intervene as necessary.

•   Record and report intervention and client's response.

Performance Checklist: Skill 6.6

Assisting with Ambulation

	S	U	NP	Comments

Assessment

1. Assess recent activity experiences (distance and tolerance).

2. Assess best time for client to ambulate relating to other schedules activities.

3. Check for handrails in hallway. Consider assitance needed.

4. Assess environment for hazards.

5. Assess client's ability and motivation to participate.

6. Assess for medications that may alter stability in ambulation.

7. Assess baseline vital signs.

Implementation

1. Use Standard Protocol.

2. Assist client to put on nonskid slippers or shoes.

3. Assist client to stand at bedside.

4. Provide client with safety belt if unstable. Consider need for additional assistance before ambulating.

5. Place IV pole on same side as site, and instruct client to push pole along while ambulating.

6. Carry or have client carry a urinary drainage bag below bladder level.

7. Take a few steps while supporting client around waist and under elbow of flexed arm nearest you. Grasp safety belt if in place.

8. Position client between you and wall, having client use handrails if available.

9. Use Completion Protocol.

	S	U	NP	Comments

Evaluation

1. Observe client ambulating. ____ ____ ____ _____

2. Evaluate client's tolerance and frequency of rest periods. ____ ____ ____ _____

3. Compare vital signs before and after ambulation and after 5 minutes of rest. ____ ____ ____ _____

4. Observe client's body alignment and balance. ____ ____ ____ _____

• Identify unexpected outcomes and intervene as necessary. ____ ____ ____ _____

• Record and report intervention and client's response. ____ ____ ____ _____

Performance Checklist: Skill 6.7

Canes, Crutches, and Walkers

	S	U	NP	Comments

Assessment

1. Review client's chart, including medical history, previous activity level, and current activity order. ___ ___ ___ _____

2. Assess client's physical readiness: vital signs and orientation to time, place, and person. ___ ___ ___ _____

3. Assess range of motion (ROM) and muscle strength or the presence of foot deformities. ___ ___ ___ _____

4. Assess client for any visual, perceptual, or sensory deficits. ___ ___ ___ _____

5. Assess environment for potential threats to client safety. Make sure floor is dry and area is well lighted. ___ ___ ___ _____

6. Assess client for discomfort. ___ ___ ___ _____

7. Assess client's understanding of technique of ambulation to be used. ___ ___ ___ _____

Implementation

1. Use Standard Protocol. ___ ___ ___ _____

Nurse Alert: Make sure the floor is clean, dry, and well-lit.

2. Prepare client for procedure.
   a. Explain reasons for exercise and demonstrate specific gait to client or caregiver.
   b. Decide with client how far to ambulate. ___ ___ ___ _____
   c. Schedule ambulation around client's other activities.
   d. Place bed in low position. ___ ___ ___ _____
   e. Help client put on well-fitting flat shoes or slippers. ___ ___ ___ _____
   f. Slowly assist client from a lying to a sitting or standing position. Assist client to stand stationary until balance is maintained. Check blood pressure as appropriate. ___ ___ ___ _____

3. Make sure that the assistive device is the appropriate height. ___ ___ ___ _____

	S	U	NP	Comments

4. Make sure assistive device has rubber tips. ___ ___ ___ _____

5. Apply safety belt if unsure of client's stability. Assist client to standing position and observe balance. If client appears weak or unsteady, return client to bed. ___ ___ ___ _____

6. Cane
   a. Client should hold cane on uninvolved side 4 to 6 inches (10-15 cm) to side of foot. Cane should extend from greater trochanter to floor. Allow approximately 15 to 30 degrees elbow flexion. ___ ___ ___ _____
   b. Assist client in ambulating with cane. (Same steps are taught whether standard or quad canes are used.) ___ ___ ___ _____
   c. Begin by placing cane on the side opposite the involved leg. ___ ___ ___ _____
   d. Place cane forward 6 to 10 inches (15-25 cm), keeping body weight on both legs. ___ ___ ___ _____
   e. Move involved leg forward, even with the cane. Begin in tripod position. Crutches are placed 6 inches (15 cm) in. ___ ___ ___ _____
   f. Advance uninvolved leg past cane. Posture should be erect. ___ ___ ___ _____
   g. Move involved leg forward, even with uninvolved leg. ___ ___ ___ _____
   h. Repeat these steps. ___ ___ ___ _____

7. Crutches
   a. Measure client for crutches.
      (1) Standing. Position crutches with crutch tips at point 4 to 6 inches (10-15 cm) to side and 4 to 6 inches in front of client's feet. Position crutch with two or three fingers between top of crutch and axilla. Instruct client to report any tingling or numbness in upper torso. ___ ___ ___ _____
      (2) Supine. Crutch pad should be three to four fingerbreadths under axilla, with crutch tips positioned 6 inches (15 cm) lateral to client's heel. ___ ___ ___ _____
      (3) Handgrip should be adjusted so that client's elbow is flexed 15 to 20 degrees using goniometer. ___ ___ ___ _____
   b. Have client stand up from a sitting position.
      (1) Move to the edge of the chair with the strong leg slightly under chair seat. ___ ___ ___ _____
      (2) Place both of the crutches in the hand on the affected side. If chair has armrests and is heavy and solid enough to avoid tipping, one armrest and both crutches may be used for bracing while rising. If the chair is

58

	S	U	NP	Comments

lightweight, both armrests should be
used for even bracing.

   (3) Push down on the crutch hand rests
while raising the body to a standing
position.

 c. Choose appropriate crutch gait.

   (1) Four-point gait

     (a) Begin in tripod position.
Crutches are placed 6 inches
(15 cm) to front and 6 inches
(15 cm) to side of each foot.
Instruct client to keep head and
neck erect, vertebrae straight,
and hips and knees extended.

     (b) Move right crutch forward 4 to
6 inches (10-15 cm).

     (c) Move left foot forward to level of
left crutch.

     (d) Move left crutch forward 4 to 6
inches.

     (e) Move right foot forward to level
of right crutch.

     (f) Repeat sequence.

   (2) Three-point gait

     (a) Begin in tripod position.

     (b) Advance both crutches and
affected leg.

     (c) Move stronger leg forward.

     (d) Repeat sequence.

   (3) Two-point gait

     (a) Begin in tripod position.

     (b) Move left crutch and right foot
forward.

     (c) Move right crutch and left foot
forward.

     (d) Repeat sequence.

   (4) Swing-to gait

     (a) Move both crutches forward

     (b) Lift and swing legs to crutches

     (c) Repeat steps.

   (5) Swing-through gait

     (a) Move both crutches forward.

     (b) Lift and swing legs through and
beyond crutches.

     (c) Repeat two previous steps.

   (6) Climbing stairs with crutches:

     (a) Begin in tripod position.

     (b) Client transfers body weight to
crutches.

     (c) Advance unaffected leg onto the
step.

     (d) Align both crutches with the
unaffected leg on the step.

	S	U	NP	Comments

(e) Repeat sequence until client reaches top of stairs. _____ _____ _____ _____

(7) Descending stairs with crutches:
(a) Begin in tripod position. _____ _____ _____ _____
(b) Transfer body weight to unaffected leg. _____ _____ _____ _____
(c) Move crutches to stair below, and instruct client to transfer body weight to crutches and move affected leg forward. _____ _____ _____ _____
(d) Move unaffected leg to stair below and align with crutches. _____ _____ _____ _____
(e) Repeat sequence until client reaches bottom step. _____ _____ _____ _____

d. Teach client to sit in a chair.
(1) Transfer both crutches to same hand and transfer weight to crutches and unaffected leg. _____ _____ _____ _____
(2) Grasp arm of chair with free hand and extend the affected leg out while lowzering into chair. _____ _____ _____ _____

8. Walker
a. Verify that upper bar of walker is slightly below client's waist. Elbows are flexed at approximately 15 to 30 degrees when standing with hands on handgrips. _____ _____ _____ _____
b. Assist client in ambulating.
(1) Have client stand in center of walker and grasp handgrips on upper bars. _____ _____ _____ _____
(2) Instruct client to lift walker, moving it 6 to 8 inches (15-20 cm) forward, all four feet of walker on the floor. Take a step forward with either foot. Then follow through with the other foot. Assist client to adjust gait according to weight-bearing ability. Instruct client not to advance the lower extremity past the front bar of the walker. _____ _____ _____ _____

9. Have client take a few steps with the assistive device being used. If client is hemiplegic (one-sided paralysis) or has hemiparesis (one-sided weakness), stand next to client's unaffected side. Support client by placing arm closest to client on safety belt or around client's waist and other arm around inferior aspect of client's upper arm. _____ _____ _____ _____

10. Take a few steps forward with client. Assess for strength and balance. _____ _____ _____ _____

11. If client becomes weak or dizzy, return to bed or chair, whichever is closer. _____ _____ _____ _____

12. Use Completion Protocol. _____ _____ _____ _____

	S	U	NP	Comments

Evaluation

1. Observe client's technique and gait while using assistive device.
   _____ _____ _____ _____

2. Inspect hands and axillae for skin irritation.
   _____ _____ _____ _____

3. Ask client to rate level of comfort.
   _____ _____ _____ _____

4. Monitor client's blood pressure, respirations, skin condition (hands and axillae), and comfort level.
   _____ _____ _____ _____

5. Ask client and family about ability to do ADLs with assistive device.
   _____ _____ _____ _____

- Identify unexpected outcomes and intervene as necessary.
   _____ _____ _____ _____

- Record and report intervention and client's response.
   _____ _____ _____ _____

Performance Checklist: Skill 7.1

Complete Bathing

	S	U	NP	Comments

Assessment

1. Assess degree of assistance needed for bathing.

2. Assess client's tolerance of activity, discomfort, shortness of breath, or chest pain with exertion.

3. Determine client's bathing preferences.

4. Identify skin changes or problems.

5. Identify limitations in client's activity or positioning.

Implementation

1. Use Standard Protocol.

2. Encourage client to assist as much as possible in bathing.

3. Provide privacy.

4. Maintain client safety.

5. Maintain warmth and comfort.

6. Incorporate the client's personal or cultural preferences for bathing.

7. Place bath blanket over client and remove top linens.

8. Remove client's gown or pajamas.
   a. Remove from unaffected side first.
   b. If IV present, remove gown from arm without IV first. Slide IV bag and tubing through sleeve and rehang. Check flow rate and regulate as necessary.
   c. If pump is used, clamp tubing and remove from pump, then proceed as in previous two steps.

9. Remove pillow and place towels under head and over the chest.

	S	U	NP	Comments

10. Wash, rinse, and dry client's face. Use plain water for the eyes. ____ ____ ____ _____
   a. Wash eyes without using soap. Dry around eyes gently. ____ ____ ____ _____
   b. Wash, rinse, and dry forehead, cheeks, nose, neck, and ears. ____ ____ ____ _____
11. Provide eye care for unconscious client. ____ ____ ____ _____
   a. Cleanse eyelids with normal saline solution. ____ ____ ____ _____
   b. Instill eye drops or ointment. ____ ____ ____ _____
   c. In absence of blink reflex, keep eyelids closed. ____ ____ ____ _____
12. Wash, rinse, and dry the upper body (arms, axillae, and chest). Apply deodorant or powder, if appropriate, to underarms. Keep only areas to be washed exposed. ____ ____ ____ _____
13. Wash, rinse, and dry lower body (abdomen, legs, and feet). Cover client, raise side rail, and change bath water and gloves. ____ ____ ____ _____

Nurse Alert: Soaking feet may be contraindicated. Avoid long, firm strokes to the legs.

14. Wash, rinse, and dry perineum, assisting client with side-lying and cleansing front to back or side to side. ____ ____ ____ _____

Nurse Alert: Perform catheter care per agency policy.

15. Provide male or female perineal care. ____ ____ ____ _____
   a. Female:
      (1) Reposition client and place waterproof pad under buttocks. Diamond-drape client. Wash, rinse, and dry groin, and wash labia majora and labia minora from pubic area toward rectum. ____ ____ ____ _____
      (2) Gently separate labia, exposing urethra and vagina, and wash from pubic area toward rectum. ____ ____ ____ _____
      (3) Rinse and dry thoroughly. Assess condition of perineal area. ____ ____ ____ _____
   b. Male:
      (1) Gently grasp shaft of penis and retract foreskin of uncircumcised client. ____ ____ ____ _____
      (2) Wash tip of penis with circular motion. Cleanse away from meatus. ____ ____ ____ _____
      (3) Cleanse shaft of penis and scrotum. Rinse and dry. ____ ____ ____ _____
16. Cover client with bath blanket. Change bath water. Remove and change gloves. ____ ____ ____ _____

	S	U	NP	Comments

17. Assist client to side-lying or prone position to wash, rinse, and dry back. Remove and dispose of gloves. ____ ____ ____ _____

18. Massage and apply lotion.
    a. Position prone or side-lying. ____ ____ ____ _____
    b. Massage in circular motions, stroking upward from buttocks using smooth, firm strokes.
    c. Knead each side of spine and around neck, avoiding bony prominences. ____ ____ ____ _____

Nurse Alert: Massaging over bony prominences may cause tissue damage.

    d. End with long strokes, telling client you are finishing. ____ ____ ____ _____
    e. Observe skin integrity. ____ ____ ____ _____

19. Apply gown or pajamas, dressing affected side first. ____ ____ ____ _____

20. Use Completion Protocol. ____ ____ ____ _____

Evaluation

1. Evaluate client's skin condition. ____ ____ ____ _____

2. Note range of motion (ROM) in joints. ____ ____ ____ _____

3. Assess vital signs if necessary. ____ ____ ____ _____

4. Observe for increasing ability to provide self-care. ____ ____ ____ _____

5. Ask client to view self in mirror. ____ ____ ____ _____

- Identify unexpected outcomes and intervene as necessary. ____ ____ ____ _____

- Record and report intervention and client's response. ____ ____ ____ _____

Performance Checklist: Procedural Guideline 7.1

Care of Dentures

	S	U	NP	Comments
1. Clean dentures for client during routine mouth care.				
2. Fill emesis basin with tepid water or, if using sink, place washcloth in bottom of sink and fill sink with an inch of water.				
3. Remove dentures. If client is unable to do this independently, apply gloves, grasp upper plate at front with thumb and index finger wrapped in gauze, and pull downward. Gently lift lower denture from jaw and rotate one side downward to remove from client's mouth. Place dentures in emesis basin or sink.				
4. Apply cleaning agent to brush and brush surface of dentures. Hold dentures close to water. Hold brush horizontally and use back-and-forth motion to cleanse biting surfaces. Use short strokes from top of denture to surfaces to clean outer and inner teeth. Hold brush vertically and use short strokes to clean inner surfaces. Hold brush horizontally and use back-and-forth motion to clean undersurface of dentures.				
5. Rinse thoroughly in tepid water.				
6. Apply a thin layer of adhesive to undersurface before inserting if desired by client.				
7. If client needs assistance with insertion, moisten upper denture and press firmly to seal it in place, then insert lower denture. Ask if dentures feel comfortable.				
8. If dentures are to be stored, keep the dentures moist and store in a secure place.				
9. Remove and discard gloves.				

Performance Checklist: Skill 7.2

Oral Care

	S	U	NP	Comments

Assessment

1. Assess presence of gag reflex with tongue blade or suction tip.

2. Inspect oral cavity.

3. Identify presence of oral problems.

Implementation

1. Use Standard Protocol.

2. Place unconscious client in side-lying position.

3. Separate upper and lower teeth gently with padded tongue blade.

4. Have suction equipment available and turned on if gag reflex is absent.

5. Clean mouth using lightly moistened brush, sponge Toothette, or 4 × 4 gauze moistened with normal saline solution.

6. Provide oral suction to remove accumulated secretions as needed.

7. Apply water-soluble jelly to lips.

8. Inform client when you have completed care.

9. Provide oral care to prevent or minimize mucositis.
   a. Provide mouth care at least four times per day.
   b. Clean mouth, brushing teeth with soft-bristled toothbrush angled at 45 degrees. Rinse with normal saline.
   c. Rinse and remove secretions.

10. See Completion Protocol.

Evaluation

1. Inspect condition of the oral cavity and client's ability to provide oral care.

	S	U	NP	Comments
2. Inspect dental surfaces for cleanliness.	___	___	___	_____
3. Observe for discomfort during care.	___	___	___	_____
4. Observe client and caregivers providing oral care.				
• Identify unexpected outcomes and intervene as necessary.	___	___	___	_____
• Record and report intervention and client's response.	___	___	___	_____

Performance Checklist: Skill 7.3

Hair Care

	S	U	NP	Comments

Assessment

1. List contraindications for exposure to moisture and limited range of motion (ROM).

2. Assess condition of hair and scalp.

3. Assess client for bleeding tendency (laboratory values PT and PTT) before shaving.

4. Assess client's ability to shave self.

Implementation

1. Use Standard Protocol.

Nurse Alert: Caution is needed if client has neck pain or neck or back injury.

2. Shampoo for client in bed (use hydrogen peroxide to remove blood)
   a. Place towel under head and brush and comb hair.
   b. Place waterproof pad under shoulders, neck, and head. Position client supine with plastic trough under head. Position spout to empty into container.
   c. Thoroughly wet, shampoo, rinse, and dry hair, taking care to avoid splashing eyes.
   d. Lather with shampoo and massage head. Rinse and towel dry. Repeat as necessary.
   e. Assist client to comfortable position and complete styling of hair.

3. Care for coarse, curly hair
   a. Shampoo hair, condition after washing. Untangle by beginning at nape of the neck.
   b. Comb small sections at a time.
   c. Lubricate hair with conditioner if needed. Use wide-toothed comb.

4. Shaving beard
   a. Assist to sitting position.
   b. Place warm, moist washcloth on face.

	S	U	NP	Comments

c. Shave carefully in direction of hair growth using short strokes and holding skin taut and razor at 45-degree angle. ___ ___ ___ _____

d. Rinse shaving cream off razor as necessary. ___ ___ ___ _____

e. Rinse and dry face. Apply aftershave if desired. Remove gloves. ___ ___ ___ _____

5. Use Completion Protocol. ___ ___ ___ _____

Evaluation

1. Offer a mirror. ___ ___ ___ _____

2. Inspect shaved skin for nicks. ___ ___ ___ _____

• Identify unexpected outcomes and intervene as necessary. ___ ___ ___ _____

• Record and report intervention and client's response. ___ ___ ___ _____

Name _____ Date _____ Instructor's Name _____

Performance Checklist: Skill 7.4

Foot and Nail Care

	S	U	NP	Comments

Assessment

1. Identify four risks for foot or nail problems.

2. Inspect all surfaces of feet, toes, and nails.

3. Assess color and warmth of feet and toes.

4. Determine client's knowledge level and ability to perform foot and nail care.

5. Ask about usual foot care practices.

6. Assess type of footwear worn by client.

Implementation

1. Use Standard Protocol.

2. Soak feet, if appropriate.
   a. Explain that soaking requires 10 to 20 minutes.

Nurse Alert: Not recommended when client has diabetes mellitus or peripheral vascular disease (PVD).

   b. Assist ambulatory client to chair with bath mat under feet, or place basin on waterproof pad on bed.
   c. Fill basin with warm water. Test temperature.
   d. Place feet in basin to soak for 10 to 20 minutes, re-warming water as necessary.
   e. Allow client to soak fingers in small basin, if desired.
   f. Soak for 10 to 20 minutes. Rewarm water as necessary.
   g. Clean under nails with orange stick. Remove hands and feet and dry thoroughly.

3. Trim or file nails straight across and evenly or file nails in presence of circulatory problems.

Nurse Alert: Referral to podiatrist indicated for patients with diabetes or severe hypertrophy. A physician's order is required for trimming nails.

	S	U	NP	Comments

4. For foot care teach client:
   a. To inspect daily
   b. To wash and soak feet daily with lukewarm water
   c. To consult physician or podiatrist to cut corns or calluses
   d. To use foot powder if feet perspire
   e. To change socks daily, or more often if wet or damp
   f. To apply lanolin or baby oil to dry areas
   g. To avoid constricting garments and crossing the legs
   h. To wear protective footwear at all times (flexible nonslip soles, closed-in toes, and adequate toe space)
   i. To wear shoes with flexible nonslip soles, closed-in toes, and adequate toe space
   j. To wash minor cuts and dry thoroughly using mild antiseptics only

5. Use Completion Protocol.

Evaluation

1. Inspect condition of client's feet.

2. Ask client to demonstrate nail care.

3. Observe ambulation after care.

• Identify unexpected outcomes and intervene as necessary.

• Record and report intervention and client's response.

Performance Checklist: Skill 7.5

Bedmaking

	S	U	NP	Comments

Assessment

1. Assess client's activity orders and ability to get out of bed.   ___ ___ ___ _____

2. Assess client's self-toileting ability and presence of wounds or drainage.   ___ ___ ___ _____

Implementation

1. Use Standard Protocol.   ___ ___ ___ _____

2. Postoperative (surgical) bed
   a. Fold top linen down from head and up from foot to center of bed.   ___ ___ ___ _____
   b. Form a triangle on one side of bed with top linen.   ___ ___ ___ _____
   c. Grasp point of the triangle and fanfold top linen.   ___ ___ ___ _____
   d. Leave bed in high position with side rails down.   ___ ___ ___ _____

3. Occupied bed
   a. Raise bed to a comfortable working height.   ___ ___ ___ _____
   b. Loosen top linens. Remove spread and blanket.   ___ ___ ___ _____
   c. Assist client to a side-lying position.   ___ ___ ___ _____
   d. Roll bottom linens toward the client.   ___ ___ ___ _____
   e. Place bottom sheet on mattress, seam side down.   ___ ___ ___ _____
   f. Cover mattress with bottom sheet. Tuck top of sheet under head of mattress.   ___ ___ ___ _____
   g. Miter corners of nonfitted sheets.   ___ ___ ___ _____
   h. Place waterproof pads and/or drawsheet on bed.   ___ ___ ___ _____
   i. Tuck remaining half of clean linens as close to client as possible.   ___ ___ ___ _____
   j. Place additional pads on top of drawsheet.   ___ ___ ___ _____
   k. Assist client to roll over linen. Raise side rail.   ___ ___ ___ _____
   l. Remove soiled linens and dispose of properly.   ___ ___ ___ _____
   m. Slide clean linen over to yourself and secure. Straighten clean linen out.   ___ ___ ___ _____
   n. Miter top corner of bottom sheet.   ___ ___ ___ _____

	S	U	NP	Comments

o. Tuck side of bottom sheet tightly along mattress, proceeding head to foot.

p. Tuck drawsheet under mattress.

q. Straighten out waterproof pads, if used.

r. Assist client to supine position. Place clean top sheet, blanket, and spread over client.

s. Slide out used top sheet or bath blanket. Cuff top sheet over blanket.

t. Make a modified mitered corner with top linens at foot of bed.

u. Loosen linens at client's feet.

v. Remove pillow, supporting client's head, and change pillowcase. Replace for comfort.

4. Use Completion Protocol.

Evaluation

1. Observe for cleanliness and absence of wrinkles.

2. Ask about level of comfort.

3. Inspect skin for irritation.

• Identify and report unexpected outcomes.

Performance Checklist: Procedural Guideline 7-2

Unoccupied Bedmaking

	S	U	NP	Comments

Assessment

1. Determine whether gloves are necessary.

2. Assess activity orders to determine that client may be out of bed for procedure. Assist client to bedside chair or recliner.

3. Lower side rails on both sides of the bed and raise bed to comfortable working height.

4. Remove soiled linen and place in laundry bag. Avoid shaking or fanning linen.

5. Reposition mattress and wipe off any moisture using a washcloth moistened in antiseptic solution. Dry thoroughly.

6. Apply all bottom linen on one side of the bed before moving to opposite side.

7. Be sure fitted sheet is placed smoothly over mattress. To apply a flat unfitted sheet, allow about 10 inches (25 cm) to hang over mattress edge. Lower hem of sheet should lie seam down, even with bottom edge of mattress. Pull remaining top portion of sheet over top edge of mattress.

8. While standing at head of bed, miter top corner of bottom sheet.

9. Tuck remaining portion of unfitted sheet under mattress.

10. Optional: Apply drawsheet, laying center fold along middle of bed lengthwise. Smooth drawsheet over mattress and tuck excess edge under mattress, keeping palms down.

11. Move to opposite side of bed and spread bottom sheet smoothly over edge of mattress from head to foot of bed.

12. Apply fitted sheet smoothly over each mattress corner. For an unfitted sheet, miter top corner of bottom sheet, making sure that corner is taut.

S   U   NP   Comments

13. Grasp remaining edge of unfitted bottom sheet and tuck tightly under mattress while moving from head to foot of bed. Smooth folded drawsheet over bottom sheet and tuck under mattress, first at middle, then at top, and then at bottom.

____   ____   ____   _____

14. If needed, apply waterproof pad between bottom sheet and drawsheet.

____   ____   ____   _____

15. Place top sheet over bed with vertical center fold lengthwise down middle of bed. Open sheet out from head to foot, being sure top edge of sheet is even with top edge of mattress.

____   ____   ____   _____

16. Make horizontal toe pleat: stand at foot of bed and fanfold sheet 2 to 4 inches (5-10 cm) across bed. Pull sheet up from bottom to make fold approximately 6 inches (15 cm) from bottom edge of mattress.

____   ____   ____   _____

17. Tuck in remaining portion of sheet under foot of mattress. Then place blanket over bed with top edge parallel to top edge of sheet and 6 to 8 inches (15-20 cm) down from edge of sheet. (Optional: Apply additional spread over bed.)

____   ____   ____   _____

18. Make cuff by turning edge of top sheet down over top edge of blanket and spread.

____   ____   ____   _____

19. Standing on one side at foot of the bed, lift mattress corner slightly with one hand and with other hand, tuck top sheet, blanket, and spread. Be sure toe pleats are not pulled out.

____   ____   ____   _____

20. Make a modified mitered corner with top sheet, blanket, and spread. After triangular fold is made, do not tuck tip of triangle.

____   ____   ____   _____

21. Go to other side of bed. Spread sheet, blanket, and spread out evenly. Make cuff with top sheet and blanket. Make modified corner at foot of bed.

____   ____   ____   _____

22. Apply clean pillowcase.

____   ____   ____   _____

23. Place call light within client's reach on bed rail or pillow and return bed to height that allows for client transfer. Assist client to bed.

____   ____   ____   _____

24. Arrange client's room. Remove and discard supplies. Wash hands.

____   ____   ____   _____

Performance Checklist: Skill 7.6

Caring for Incontinent Clients

	S	U	NP	Comments

Assessment

1. Assess frequency of episodes of incontinence; observe for a pattern.

2. Assess amount with each occurrence.

3. Assess episodes related to specific events (coughing, sneezing, exercise).

4. Assess condition of skin in perineal area.

5. Assess fluid intake and characteristics of urine.

Implementation

1. Use Standard Protocol.

2. Provide client with opportunity to use bathroom, bedpan, or commode.

3. Maintain record of continent and incontinent periods.

4. Apply gloves. Turn client to supine position with legs abducted.
   a. Female: Wash labia with soap and warm water. Gently retract labia from thigh and wash groin from perineum to rectum.
   b. Male: Wash penis beginning with urinary meatus, retracting foreskin if client is uncircumcised. Gently cleanse shaft of penis and scrotum, washing all skin folds. Return foreskin to natural position.

5. Turn client to side and continue cleansing. Dry thoroughly.

6. Place absorbent underpad under client.

7. Expose perineal area to air whenever possible. Apply skin barrier or sealant, or vitamin A–enriched cream.

8. Provide pads or briefs to ambulatory clients.

9. Remove and dispose of gloves.

	S	U	NP	Comments

10. Use Completion Protocol. ___ ___ ___ _____

Evaluation

1. Evaluate amount of incontinent episodes in relation to events of elimination. ___ ___ ___ _____

2. Observe effectiveness of absorbent pads or garments. ___ ___ ___ _____

3. Continue to observe and protect skin. ___ ___ ___ _____

- Identify unexpected outcomes and intervene as necessary. ___ ___ ___ _____

- Record and report intervention and client's response. ___ ___ ___ _____

Performance Checklist: Skill 8.1

Feeding Dependent Clients

	S	U	NP	Comments

Assessment

1. Assess client's level of consciousness, ability to participate, mobility or activity orders, and physical limitations. ___ ___ ___ _____

2. Assess need for toileting, hand washing, and oral care before feeding. ___ ___ ___ _____

3. Determine client's food tolerance and cultural or religious preferences. ___ ___ ___ _____

4. Measure client's weight and determine special diet requirements. ___ ___ ___ _____

5. Assess pertinent laboratory values. ___ ___ ___ _____

Implementation

1. Use Standard Protocol. ___ ___ ___ _____

2. Provide toileting and hand washing before feeding. ___ ___ ___ _____

3. Offer oral care before meal.

4. Check environment for distractions.

5. Position client appropriately (sitting in chair, high Fowler's position, or side-lying). ___ ___ ___ _____

6. Assist client in setting up meal tray. ___ ___ ___ _____

7. Place adaptive utensils on tray and instruct client in their use. ___ ___ ___ _____

8. Identify food location on plate for visually impaired client. ___ ___ ___ _____

9. Pace feeding time to avoid client fatigue. Interact with client during meal. ___ ___ ___ _____

10. Assist client with washing hands and repositioning.

11. Monitor client's I&O and calorie count. ___ ___ ___ _____

12. Use Completion Protocol. ___ ___ ___ _____

	S	U	NP	Comments

Evaluation

1. Monitor body weight. ___ ___ ___ _____

2. Monitor laboratory values. ___ ___ ___ _____

3. Observe self-feeding abilities. ___ ___ ___ _____

4. Observe choking cough or gag. ___ ___ ___ _____

5. Observe use of adaptive utensils. ___ ___ ___ _____

6. Observe food left on tray. ___ ___ ___ _____

• Identify unexpected outcomes and intervene as necessary. ___ ___ ___ _____

• Record and report intervention and client's response. ___ ___ ___ _____

Name _____ Date _____ Instructor's Name _____

Performance Checklist: Skill 8.2

Assisting Clients with Impaired Swallowing

	S	U	NP	Comments

Assessment

1. Assess client's level of consciousness, drooling, and speech. ___ ___ ___ _____

2. Assess lung sounds and ability to cough on request. ___ ___ ___ _____

3. Determine presence of gag reflex and swallowing reflex. ___ ___ ___ _____

4. Assess client's weight and pertinent laboratory values. ___ ___ ___ _____

Implementation

1. Use Standard Protocol. ___ ___ ___ _____

2. Position client upright with head slightly flexed forward. ___ ___ ___ _____

3. Reduce environmental distractions. ___ ___ ___ _____

4. Add thickener to thin liquids or start with pureed foods. ___ ___ ___ _____

5. Place ½ to 1 tsp on unaffected side of mouth. ___ ___ ___ _____

6. Place hand on throat to gently palpate swallowing as it occurs. ___ ___ ___ _____

7. Provide verbal coaching while feeding.
   a. Open your mouth. ___ ___ ___ _____
   b. Feel the food in your mouth. ___ ___ ___ _____
   c. Chew and taste the food. ___ ___ ___ _____
   d. Raise your tongue to the roof of your mouth. ___ ___ ___ _____
   e. Think about swallowing. ___ ___ ___ _____
   f. Close your mouth and swallow. ___ ___ ___ _____
   g. Swallow again. ___ ___ ___ _____
   h. Cough to clear your airway. ___ ___ ___ _____

8. Observe for coughing, gagging, choking; suction as needed. ___ ___ ___ _____

9. Provide rest periods as needed. ___ ___ ___ _____

10. Maintain upright position for 15 to 30 minutes after feeding. ___ ___ ___ _____

11. Provide mouth care after meals. ___ ___ ___ _____

	S	U	NP	Comments

12. Advance diet to thicker foods, then to thin liquids as tolerated.   ____ ____ ____ _____

13. Use Completion Protocol.   ____ ____ ____ _____

Evaluation

1. Observe contents of client's mouth during meal.   ____ ____ ____ _____

2. Evaluate ability of client to safely swallow food.   ____ ____ ____ _____

3. Presence of choking or coughing.   ____ ____ ____ _____

4. Determine client's intake and output.   ____ ____ ____ _____

5. Monitor client's weight.   ____ ____ ____ _____

6. Monitor pertinent laboratory values.   ____ ____ ____ _____

• Identify unexpected outcomes and intervene as necessary.   ____ ____ ____ _____

• Record and report intervention and client's response.   ____ ____ ____ _____

Performance Checklist: Procedural Guideline 8-1

Standing Height and Weight on Platform or Chair Scale

	S	U	NP	Comments

Implementation

1. Use Standard Protocol.

2. Assess client's ability to bear weight and safely stand on a scale.

3. Apply gloves. Empty any pouches or drainage devices.

4. Weigh client.
   a. Platform or chair scale
      (1) Place platform or chair scale at client's bedside.
      (2) Balance and calibrate the scale.
      (3) Ask client to step onto platform scale and remain still, or assist client to sit on chair scale.
      (4) Adjust balance on scale until it is in the middle of mark or until digital scale displays reading.
      (5) Swing the metal rod attached to the back of the scale over the crown of the head with client standing erect and without wearing shoes.
      (6) Measure height in inches or centimeters.
   b. Bed scale
      (1) Place sling with same type and amount of linen and client's gown on arms of scale.
      (2) Calibrate bed scale for sling, linens, and client's gown.
      (3) With nurse on each side of bed, roll client onto side. Place sling under client.
      (4) Attach scale and elevate until clear of bed.
      (5) Instruct client to remain still.
      (6) Read digital weight on scale.
      (7) Lower client onto bed, roll over stretcher, then remove stretcher and scale from client's bed.

		S	U	NP	Comments
5.	Compare weight obtained with previous measurement.	___	___	___	_____
6.	Record weight on appropriate form.	___	___	___	_____
7.	Use Completion Protocol.	___	___	___	_____

Performance Checklist: Skill 9.1

Monitoring Intake and Output

	S	U	NP	Comments

Assessment

1. Identify medications that may alter urine output.

2. Monitor hematocrit.

3. Weigh client daily (same time, scale, and clothes).

4. Assess signs and symptoms of fluid excess or deficit.

5. Assess client's and family's knowledge of and ability to assist with intake and output measurement.

Implementation

1. Use Standard Protocol.

2. Explain purpose of intake and output.

3. Measure and record all fluid intake.
   a. Liquids with meals including gelatin, custards, ice cream, Popsicles, and sherbet. Ice chips are 50% of measured volume
   b. Liquid medications
   c. Tube feedings (enteral nutrition)
   d. IV fluids

4. Instruct client and family to notify nurse to empty urinal or bedpan after each use.

5. Apply gloves to empty urinary output from Foley catheter.

Nurse Alert: Hourly urine output <30 ml/hr should be reported.

6. Observe characteristics of urine output.

7. Measure and record all output, including urine and drainage from all sources.
   a. Nasogastric suction
   b. Chest tube drainage
   c. Jackson-Pratt or Hemovac drains
   d. Emesis

	S	U	NP	Comments

8. Remove gloves. ___ ___ ___ _____

9. Use Completion Protocol. ___ ___ ___ _____

Evaluation

1. Observe amount and characteristics of urine. ___ ___ ___ _____

2. Calculate client's intake and output every shift and total for 24 hours. ___ ___ ___ _____

3. Monitor relevant laboratory results. ___ ___ ___ _____

4. Compare daily weights >2% in 48 hours. ___ ___ ___ _____

- Identify unexpected outcomes and intervene as necessary. ___ ___ ___ _____

- Record and report intervention and client's response. ___ ___ ___ _____

Performance Checklist: Skill 9.2

Providing a Bedpan and Urinal

	S	U	NP	Comments

Assessment

1. Check order for bed rest.

2. Use common language when talking to client to promote understanding.

3. Assess elimination pattern.

4. Assess length and extent of immobility.

5. Assess client's ability to assist, lift hips, and turn.

6. Determine need for urine or stool specimen collection.

7. Assess I&O.

8. Assess dietary intake (fiber and fluids).

9. Determine extent and location of discomfort.

10. Assess bowel sounds, palpate abdomen, and assess ability to pass flatus.

Implementation

1. Use Standard Protocol.

2. Provide bedpan.
   a. Lower head of bed and assist client to roll toward you.
   b. Raise side rail.
   c. Go to opposite side of bed and place warmed bedpan under client's buttocks.
   d. Press bedpan firmly down onto mattress. Assist client to roll onto bedpan.
   e. Place bedpan under client directly if client is able to lift self.
   f. Raise head of bed at least 30 to 40 degrees, unless contraindicated.
   g. Raise side rail and place call bell and toilet paper within reach. Discard gloves. Provide privacy.
   h. Lower head of bed and side rail when client is finished. Assist client to roll away from you while securing bedpan.
   i. Assist client with cleaning as necessary.

	S	U	NP	Comments

j. Provide opportunity for client to wash
hands. ___ ___ ___ _____

k. Measure contents and dispose into toilet. ___ ___ ___ _____

l. Rinse bedpan and store appropriately
(in bathroom or covered on chair seat). ___ ___ ___ _____

m. Discard gloves. ___ ___ ___ _____

**Nurse Alert: Note color and appearance of urine
and stool.**

3. Provide urinal for male client.
   a. Position client with head elevated or
   standing. ___ ___ ___ _____

   b. Assist client as needed to have penis
   placed into urinal. ___ ___ ___ _____

   c. Instruct client to notify caregiver each
   time urinal is used. Measure contents for
   I&O, then empty contents into toilet. ___ ___ ___ _____

   d. Place urinal within client's reach on side
   rail. ___ ___ ___ _____

   e. Discard gloves. ___ ___ ___ _____

4. Use Completion Protocol. ___ ___ ___ _____

Evaluation

1. Determine client's ability to assist. ___ ___ ___ _____

2. Evaluate characteristics of stool. ___ ___ ___ _____

3. Observe characteristics of urine. ___ ___ ___ _____

4. Observe skin integrity. ___ ___ ___ _____

- Identify unexpected outcomes and intervene
as necessary. ___ ___ ___ _____

- Record and report intervention and client's
response. ___ ___ ___ _____

Name _____ Date _____ Instructor's Name _____

Performance Checklist: Skill 9.3

Applying an External Catheter

	S	U	NP	Comments

Assessment

1. Assess urinary elimination patterns, ability to urinate voluntarily, and continence. ___ ___ ___ _____

2. Assess mental status of client and knowledge of treatment. ___ ___ ___ _____

3. Assess condition of penis. ___ ___ ___ _____

Implementation

1. Use Standard Protocol. ___ ___ ___ _____

2. Assist client to supine position, covering upper torso and lower extremities. ___ ___ ___ _____

3. Prepare urinary drainage system. Clamp drainage exit port. Secure bag to bed frame with tubing between bed and side rails. Prepare leg bag, if necessary. ___ ___ ___ _____

4. Wash, rinse, and dry penis thoroughly with warm soapy water. ___ ___ ___ _____

5. Clip hair at base of penis if necessary. ___ ___ ___ _____

6. Apply skin preparation to penis and allow to dry. ___ ___ ___ _____

7. Apply self-adhesive external catheter.
   a. Plastic collar positions inner flap for application. ___ ___ ___ _____
   b. Pinch catheter closed and place against glans so that tip protrudes $1/4$ inch into opening. ___ ___ ___ _____
   c. Grasp penis with nondominant hand and unroll catheter up shaft of penis with other hand. ___ ___ ___ _____

Nurse Alert: Do not push collar onto penis.

   d. Gently squeeze catheter to adhere sheath to skin. Pinch wrinkles to seal openings. ___ ___ ___ _____

8. Apply external catheter without adhesive.
   a. Apply sheath to penis as in step 7.
   b. Allow 1 to 2 inches of space between tip of penis and end of catheter. ___ ___ ___ _____

	S	U	NP	Comments

c. Encircle penis with strip of elastic adhesive kept only in contact with sheath.   ____ ____ ____ _____

Nurse Alert: Do not use standard tape or Velcro, which can alter circulation and cause necrosis.

9. Connect drainage tubing to end of catheter.   ____ ____ ____ _____

10. Secure tubing so that it is not twisted or looped. Discard gloves.   ____ ____ ____ _____

11. Remove catheter for 30 minutes every 24 hours to cleanse and inspect skin.   ____ ____ ____ _____

12. Use Completion Protocol.   ____ ____ ____ _____

Evaluation

1. Observe urinary output every 4 hours.   ____ ____ ____ _____

2. Remove sheath and inspect penile skin at least daily and when external catheter is reapplied.   ____ ____ ____ _____

3. Assess condition of skin and circulation to penis 1 hour after application, then every 4 hours.   ____ ____ ____ _____

• Identify unexpected outcomes and intervene as necessary.   ____ ____ ____ _____

• Record and report intervention and client's response.   ____ ____ ____ _____

Performance Checklist: Skill 9.4

Administering an Enema

	S	U	NP	Comments

Assessment

1. Assess last bowel movement and presence or absence of bowel sounds. _____ _____ _____ _____

2. Assess ability to control external sphincter by performing rectal exam. _____ _____ _____ _____

3. Determine presence of hemorrhoids. _____ _____ _____ _____

4. Assess abdominal pain. _____ _____ _____ _____

5. Assess client's understanding of procedure. _____ _____ _____ _____

6. Assess client's mobility status. _____ _____ _____ _____

Implementation

1. Use Standard Protocol. _____ _____ _____ _____

2. Fill enema bag with 750 to 1000 ml warm tap water. Check temperature of water. Fill tubing with solution, removing air, and clamp. _____ _____ _____ _____

3. Add castile soap to water if ordered. _____ _____ _____ _____

4. Assist client to left side-lying (Sims') position with right knee flexed. Encourage to remain in position until procedure is completed. _____ _____ _____ _____

Nurse Alert: Clients with minimal sphincter control may require a bed pan.

5. Place waterproof pad under hips and buttocks. _____ _____ _____ _____

6. Cover client with bath blanket, exposing only rectal area. _____ _____ _____ _____

7. Ensure that toilet, bedpan, or commode is available. _____ _____ _____ _____

8. Administer enema in disposable prepackaged container.
   a. Remove plastic cap from rectal tip, applying more lubricant to cap if needed. _____ _____ _____ _____
   b. Gently separate buttocks and locate anus. Instruct client to take deep breaths through mouth. _____ _____ _____ _____
   c. Insert lubricated tip into rectum 3 to 4 inches (adult). _____ _____ _____ _____

	S	U	NP	Comments

d. Squeeze bottle continuously until all fluid is expelled. ___ ___ ___ _____

9. Administer in standard enema bag.
   a. Lubricate 3 to 4 inches of tip of tubing. ___ ___ ___ _____
   b. Gently separate buttocks and locate anus. ___ ___ ___ _____
   c. Insert tip of tube slowly, pointing tip toward umbilicus, for 3 to 4 inches (adult) past internal sphincter. ___ ___ ___ _____
   d. Hold tubing until fluid is instilled. ___ ___ ___ _____
   e. With container at hip level, open clamp and begin instillation. ___ ___ ___ _____
   f. Raise height of container to 12 to 18 inches above anus and hang on IV pole. ___ ___ ___ _____
   g. Lower height of container if client experiences cramping or fluid escapes around tube. ___ ___ ___ _____
   h. Clamp tubing after solution instilled and inform client that tubing will be removed. Gently withdraw tube. ___ ___ ___ _____

10. Explain to client that a feeling of distention is expected. Ask client to retain solution as long as possible (5-10 minutes). ___ ___ ___ _____

11. Discard enema container and tubing, or rinse if to be reused. ___ ___ ___ _____

12. Assist client to use bathroom, bedpan, or commode. ___ ___ ___ _____

13. Instruct clients with history of cardiovascular disease to exhale during defecation (Valsalva maneuver can cause cardiac arrest). ___ ___ ___ _____

14. Instruct client to call for nurse to inspect results before discarding. Observe character of feces and solution. ___ ___ ___ _____

15. Assist client with perineal care as necessary. ___ ___ ___ _____

16. Discard gloves. ___ ___ ___ _____

17. Use Completion Protocol. ___ ___ ___ _____

Evaluation

1. Evaluate results of enema (decreased abdominal discomfort; palpate abdomen). ___ ___ ___ _____

2. Observe characteristics of stool and fluid. ___ ___ ___ _____

• Identify unexpected outcomes and intervene as necessary. ___ ___ ___ _____

• Record and report intervention and client's response. ___ ___ ___ _____

Name _____ Date _____ Instructor's Name _____

Performance Checklist: Skill 9.5

Catheter Care

	S	U	NP	Comments

Assessment

1. Assess urethral meatus and surrounding tissues. ___ ___ ___ _____

2. Assess characteristics of urine. ___ ___ ___ _____

3. Assess for presence of pain or discomfort in lower abdomen. ___ ___ ___ _____

4. Monitor client's temperature. ___ ___ ___ _____

5. Monitor client's fluid intake. ___ ___ ___ _____

6. Assess client's understanding of procedure. ___ ___ ___ _____

Implementation

1. Use Standard Protocol. ___ ___ ___ _____

2. Position client comfortably and cover with bath blanket, exposing only perineal area.
   a. Position female in dorsal recumbent position.
   b. Position male in supine position. ___ ___ ___ _____

3. Place waterproof pad under client. ___ ___ ___ _____

4. Apply gloves. Provide routine perineal care. ___ ___ ___ _____

5. Hold catheter securely near the meatus with gloved nondominant hand. Using a clean washcloth, soap, and water, take the dominant hand and wipe in a circular motion along the length of the catheter for about 4 inches (10 cm). Avoid placing tension on or pulling the catheter tubing. ___ ___ ___ _____

6. Replace, if necessary, the anchor device used to secure the tubing to the client's leg or abdomen. ___ ___ ___ _____

7. Check drainage tubing and bag to ensure that:
   a. Tubing is not looped or above the level of the bladder.
   b. Tubing is coiled and secured.
   c. Tubing is not kinked or clamped.
   d. Collection bag is positioned appropriately on bed frame. ___ ___ ___ _____

	S	U	NP	Comments

8. Empty collection bag as necessary or at least every 8 hours. _____ _____ _____ _____

9. Use Completion Protocol. _____ _____ _____ _____

Evaluation

1. Observe amount and characteristics of urine. _____ _____ _____ _____

2. Inspect the catheter insertion site for secretions and encrustations. _____ _____ _____ _____

3. Monitor the client's temperature. _____ _____ _____ _____

4. Ask client about feelings of discomfort or burning.

• Identify unexpected outcomes and intervene as necessary. _____ _____ _____ _____

• Record and report intervention and client's response. _____ _____ _____ _____

Name _____ Date _____ Instructor's Name _____

Performance Checklist: Skill 10.1

Comfort Measures that Promote Sleep

	S	U	NP	Comments

Assessment

1. Assess discomfort (onset, precipitating factors, quality, region, severity). ____ ____ ____ _____

2. Determine client's normal sleep pattern and any problems. ____ ____ ____ _____

3. Describe the sleep problem experienced. ____ ____ ____ _____

4. Identify medications that may influence sleep patterns. ____ ____ ____ _____

5. Identify illnesses or conditions that can alter sleep. ____ ____ ____ _____

6. Identify five indications of sleep apnea. ____ ____ ____ _____

Implementation

1. Use Standard Protocol. ____ ____ ____ _____

2. Promote usual bedtime routines. ____ ____ ____ _____

3. Offer bedtime snack. Suggest avoiding caffeine at bedtime. ____ ____ ____ _____

4. Schedule diuretics early in the day. Decrease fluid intake at bedtime. ____ ____ ____ _____

5. Teach client to reduce or eliminate physical activities 2 hours before bedtime. ____ ____ ____ _____

6. Encourage client to avoid alcohol before bedtime. ____ ____ ____ _____

7. Make sure client's gown and linens are clean and dry. ____ ____ ____ _____

8. Provide cutaneous stimulation, such as a massage or warm bath or cold compress. ____ ____ ____ _____

9. Assist client to comfortable position. Support body parts. ____ ____ ____ _____

10. Raise side rails and place call bell within reach. Use fall precaution guidelines, if indicated. ____ ____ ____ _____

11. Reduce environmental noise. ____ ____ ____ _____

12. Provide indirect light. ____ ____ ____ _____

	S	U	NP	Comments

13. Schedule assessments and treatments to minimize disturbance. ___ ___ ___ _____

14. Use Completion Protocol. ___ ___ ___ _____

Evaluation

1. Ask to rate discomfort level (0-10). ___ ___ ___ _____

2. Observe for sleep in 30 minutes and hourly thereafter. ___ ___ ___ _____

3. Ask to describe methods used to promote sleep. ___ ___ ___ _____

4. Assess perception of feeling rested. ___ ___ ___ _____

• Identify unexpected outcomes and intervene as necessary. ___ ___ ___ _____

• Record and report intervention and client's response. ___ ___ ___ _____

Performance Checklist: Skill 10-2

Relaxation Techniques

	S	U	NP	Comments

Assessment

1. Assess character of client's discomfort.

2. Assess verbal and nonverbal discomfort.

3. Observe for signs of physical or psychological distress.

4. Observe social interactions.

5. Assess for signs of anxiety or stress.

6. Determine whether client has bleeding tendency or is receiving anticoagulants.

7. Assess types of activities client uses to promote relaxation.

8. Assess client's willingness to receive non-pharmacologic pain relief measures.

9. Assess for spiritual concerns or distress.

Implementation

1. Use Standard Protocol.

2. Remove environmental distractions.

3. Distraction
   a. Ask client to close eyes or focus on an object.
   b. Apply activities determined in assessment to direct attention away from discomfort.

4. Progressive muscle relaxation

Nurse Alert: Teach client only if not in acute distress.

   a. Assist client to position of comfort, with body well supported sitting or lying down.
   b. Apply light sheet or blanket.
   c. Instruct to close eyes, relax, and breathe slowly and deeply.
   d. Instruct to follow cues for relaxing.
   e. Begin series of alternately tightening and relaxing each muscle group (head to toe).
   f. Ask client to enjoy relaxed feeling and allow mind to drift. Ask to breathe deeply.

g. Instruct client to perform the following, relaxing after each, and repeating each step two times on both sides of the body. ____ ____ ____ _____

  (1) Arm reaching, eye squinting, jaw tightening, moving shoulder to earlobe, abdominal muscle tightening, hips and buttocks tightening, pressing legs into the mattress, pointing and stretching toes, legs, and feet, and entire body relaxation ____ ____ ____ _____

h. Return to muscle group if tightening occurs in that group. ____ ____ ____ _____

i. Explain that client may feel tingling, heaviness, floating, or warmth. ____ ____ ____ _____

j. Ask client to continue slow, deep breaths. ____ ____ ____ _____

k. Instruct to inhale, exhale, then move around slowly after relaxation is completed. ____ ____ ____ _____

5. Guided imagery
  a. Assist to position of comfort. ____ ____ ____ _____

  b. Sit close and speak in soft, calm voice. ____ ____ ____ _____

  c. Have client breathe in slow, rhythmic manner. ____ ____ ____ _____

  d. Suggest relaxation. ____ ____ ____ _____

  e. Direct through imagery using pleasant experiences. ____ ____ ____ _____

  f. Use direct imagery. ____ ____ ____ _____

  g. Encourage client to practice imagery. ____ ____ ____ _____

  h. Have client continue deep, slow rhythmic breathing. ____ ____ ____ _____

  i. End the experience by reinforcing a sense of relaxation. ____ ____ ____ _____

6. Massage
  a. Adjust bed to comfortable working height and lower side rail. ____ ____ ____ _____

  b. Assist client to comfortable lying or sitting position. ____ ____ ____ _____

Nurse Alert: Clients with respiratory difficulty may lie on side with head elevated.

  c. Turn on soft, pleasing music. ____ ____ ____ _____

  d. Drape client to expose only area for massage. ____ ____ ____ _____

  e. Warm lotion in hands, for use after head and scalp massage. ____ ____ ____ _____

  f. Select body part to be massaged. Massage each part for 3 minutes. ____ ____ ____ _____

Nurse Alert: Clients who are heavily medicated or unable to communicate need very gentle massage.

  g. Select stroke technique to use. ____ ____ ____ _____

  h. Encourage client to breathe slowly and deeply. ____ ____ ____ _____

	S	U	NP	Comments

i. Make contact with skin first. ___ ___ ___ _____

j. Massage head and scalp. Do not use lotion. Stimulate scalp and temples. ___ ___ ___ _____

k. Massage hands and arms. Glide hands over arms. Massage each finger. Knead arm muscles. ___ ___ ___ _____

l. Massage neck. Support neck and knead muscles on each side. ___ ___ ___ _____

m. Massage back. Stroke upward from buttocks to shoulders. Knead muscles of upper back and shoulders. ___ ___ ___ _____

Nurse Alert: Be certain to massage muscular regions, not bones of spine. Avoid bruised, swollen, or inflamed areas.

n. Massage feet, avoiding bunions or other sensitive areas. Use circular motion around ankle and feet. ___ ___ ___ _____

o. Instruct client to relax and breathe slowly. Remove excess oil. ___ ___ ___ _____

7. Use Completion Protocol. ___ ___ ___ _____

Evaluation

1. Evaluate level of comfort and relaxation. ___ ___ ___ _____

2. Inspect physiological and behavioral responses. ___ ___ ___ _____

3. Observe client's performance of techniques. ___ ___ ___ _____

4. Ask client to demonstrate techniques at a time of low stress. ___ ___ ___ _____

• Identify unexpected outcomes and intervene as necessary. ___ ___ ___ _____

• Record and report intervention and client's response. ___ ___ ___ _____

Performance Checklist: Skill 11.1

Nonpharmacological Pain Management

	S	U	NP	Comments

Assessment

1. Identify factors that cause discomfort and pain.
2. Assess client's perception of the discomfort and pain.
3. Assess client's culturally determined beliefs about pain.
4. Assess sensation of pain.
5. Perform physical assessment at site of pain.
6. Assess physiological and psychological responses to pain.
7. Assess behavioral responses to pain.
8. Obtain pain intensity rating from primary caregiver if client is cognitively impaired.
9. Assess environmental factors that may influence the pain experience.
10. Determine what relieves the discomfort or what the client believes will help.
11. Consider physician's order for activity, intake, and medications.

Implementation

1. Use Standard Protocol.
2. Teach client how to use pain intensity scale.
3. Set pain intensity goal with client.
4. Remove or reduce painful stimuli.
   a. Reposition client.
   b. Apply gloves. Change dressings if wet or constricting.
   c. Reapply or adjust equipment as needed.
5. Reduce or eliminate factors that increase the pain experience.
   a. Relate acceptance and acknowledge the reality of the pain experience.
   b. Explain the cause of pain (if known), providing accurate information.

	S	U	NP	Comments

6. Assist client to splint painful area using firm pressure over a bath blanket or pillow during coughing, deep breathing, and turning. ____ ____ ____ _____

7. Massage painful area gently or firmly. ____ ____ ____ _____

Nurse Alert: Do not massage areas with abnormal reactive hyperemia or in the presence of bleeding tendencies.

8. Encourage relaxation using imagery, progressive relaxation, or deep rhythmic breathing. ____ ____ ____ _____

9. Direct client's attention to something else that increases pain tolerance. ____ ____ ____ _____

10. Reposition client for comfort and leave room clean and pleasant. ____ ____ ____ _____

11. Use Completion Protocol. ____ ____ ____ _____

Evaluation

1. Ask client to rate pain intensity. ____ ____ ____ _____

2. Evaluate PQRST aspects of pain. ____ ____ ____ _____

3. Continue to evaluate client's level of comfort and objective and subjective responses to interventions. ____ ____ ____ _____

• Identify unexpected outcomes and intervene as necessary. ____ ____ ____ _____

• Record and report intervention and client's response. ____ ____ ____ _____

Performance Checklist: Skill 11.2

Pharmacological Pain Management

	S	U	NP	Comments
Assessment				
1. Perform complete pain assessment.	___	___	___	_____
2. Determine time of administration of previously administered medications, including dose, length of time, and degree of relief experienced.	___	___	___	_____
3. Determine whether client has allergies to medications.	___	___	___	_____
4. Determine analgesics prescribed, route, and frequency.	___	___	___	_____
Implementation				
1. Use Standard Protocol.	___	___	___	_____
2. Review six rights of administration.	___	___	___	_____

Nurse Alert: Extended release opioids may not be crushed for administration via gastrostomy or jejunostomy tubes.

	S	U	NP	Comments
3. Administer analgesics.				
a. As soon as pain occurs				
b. Before it increases in severity	___	___	___	_____
c. Before pain-producing procedures or activities				
d. As routinely scheduled	___	___	___	_____
4. Include nonpharmacological pain control measures in addition to analgesics.	___	___	___	_____
5. Identify expected time for peak effects and usual duration of action of analgesics.	___	___	___	_____
6. Coordinate nursing care measures to maximize effectiveness.	___	___	___	_____
7. Monitor for adverse effects.				
8. Remove and dispose of gloves.	___	___	___	_____
9. Use Completion Protocol.	___	___	___	_____

	S	U	NP	Comments

Evaluation

1. Evaluate client's level of comfort using a pain scale at appropriate intervals. ___ ___ ___ _____

2. Evaluate PQRST aspects of pain. ___ ___ ___ _____

3. Continue client's position, mobility, relaxation, and ability to rest and sleep. ___ ___ ___ _____

• Identify unexpected outcomes and intervene as necessary. ___ ___ ___ _____

• Record and report intervention and client's response. ___ ___ ___ _____

Performance Checklist: Skill 11.3

Patient-Controlled Analgesia

	S	U	NP	Comments

Assessment

1. Check physician's orders for prescribed medication, dosage, and lockout settings. Verify that client is not allergic to prescribed medication. ____ ____ ____ _____

2. Verify patency of the IV site and compatibility with the solution currently infusing. ____ ____ ____ _____

3. Determine client's physical ability to manipulate PCA device and cognitive ability to understand directions. ____ ____ ____ _____

4. Assess baseline pain intensity, sedation level, and respiratory status. ____ ____ ____ _____

5. Assess if client has history of sleep apnea. ____ ____ ____ _____

Implementation

1. Use Standard Protocol. ____ ____ ____ _____

2. Teach the client about PCA before the therapy is initiated. ____ ____ ____ _____
    a. Advantages ____ ____ ____ _____
    b. Use of control button ____ ____ ____ _____
    c. Lockout feature ____ ____ ____ _____
    d. Possible side effects ____ ____ ____ _____
    e. To notify nurse if unable to control pain ____ ____ ____ _____

3. Prepare medication for infusion.
    a. Attach prefilled medication reservoir to pump device. ____ ____ ____ _____
    b. Prime the unit. ____ ____ ____ _____
    c. Adjust PCA to reflect physician's orders and lock settings. ____ ____ ____ _____

4. Transport equipment to client's room and plug into electrical outlet. ____ ____ ____ _____

5. Verify client identity by checking identification band and asking client to state name. ____ ____ ____ _____

6. Attach PCA tubing to client's IV tubing.
    a. Open all clamps. ____ ____ ____ _____
    b. Start pump. ____ ____ ____ _____

		S	U	NP	Comments

c. Be sure maintenance IV rate is at least 50 ml/hour.

d. Place control device within easy reach of client.

7. Reinforce previous teaching of proper use of PCA pump. Assist client to self-administer initial dose by pressing button.

8. Encourage client to self-administer medication without delay whenever discomfort is felt.

9. Instruct family to support and assist client, but not to administer medication independently while client is sleeping.

10. Involve client in planning care activities.

11. To discontinue PCA:
   a. Obtain necessary PCA information from pump.
   b. Turn pump off.
   c. Disconnect PCA tubing from IV line.
   d. Dispose of remaining opioid appropriately.

12. Use Completion Protocol.

Nuse Alert: If pump is discontinued with opioid remaining, waste must be witnessed and documented.

Evaluation

1. Evaluate client's ability to manipulate control button.

2. Observe ability to cooperate and respond to instructions.

3. Ask client to rate pain using pain scale.

4. Observe respiratory rate and depth and level of consciousness regularly.

Nurse Alert: Do not increase demand or basal dose and decrease the interval time simultaneously.

• Identify unexpected outcomes and intervene as necessary.

• Record and report intervention and client's response.

Performance Checklist: Skill 11.4

Epidural Analgesia

	S	U	NP	Comments

Assessment

1. Assess client's pain. _____ _____ _____ _____

2. Assess client's nonverbal response. _____ _____ _____ _____

3. Assess sedation level of client, including level of consciousness (LOC), to establish a baseline before first dose. _____ _____ _____ _____

4. Check rate, depth, and pattern of respirations to establish a baseline. _____ _____ _____ _____

5. Check blood pressure to establish a baseline. _____ _____ _____ _____

6. Assess mobility and motor and sensory function before assisting client into or out of bed. _____ _____ _____ _____

7. Check to see if epidural catheter is secured to client's skin. _____ _____ _____ _____

8. Assess condition of skin. _____ _____ _____ _____

9. Assess epidural catheter insertion site for redness, warmth, tenderness, swelling, and drainage. _____ _____ _____ _____

10. If continuous infusion, check infusion pump for proper calibration and operation to ensure client will obtain prescribed analgesic dose. _____ _____ _____ _____

11. If continuous infusion, check patency of IV tubing. _____ _____ _____ _____

12. Check client's history of drug allergies. _____ _____ _____ _____

Implementation

1. Use Standard Protocol. _____ _____ _____ _____

2. Verify client's identity. _____ _____ _____ _____

3. Review six rights of medication administration. _____ _____ _____ _____

4. Apply gloves. Prepare and administer bolus injection.
   a. Attach "epidural line" label close to injection cap on epidural catheter. _____ _____ _____ _____

	S	U	NP	Comments

b. Using a large syringe, draw up prediluted preservative-free narcotic solution through a filter needle. ___ ___ ___ _____

c. Change from filter needle to regular 20-gauge needle. ___ ___ ___ _____

d. Clean injection cap with povidone-iodine (do not use alcohol). ___ ___ ___ _____

e. Dry the injection cap with sterile 2 × 2 gauze. ___ ___ ___ _____

f. Insert needle or syringe (needleless system) into injection cap. Aspirate. ___ ___ ___ _____

g. If less than 1 ml clear fluid returns, inject drug slowly. ___ ___ ___ _____

h. Remove needle from injection cap. ___ ___ ___ _____

i. Dispose of uncapped needle and syringe in sharps container. ___ ___ ___ _____

Nurse Alert: Keep an ampule of naloxone (Narcan) at the beside to counteract severe respiratory depression.

5. Apply gloves. Administer continuous infusion.

   a. Attach "epidural line" label to IV tubing connected to epidural catheter. Use tubing without Y ports. ___ ___ ___ _____

   b. Attach container of diluted preservative-free narcotic to infusion pump tubing, and prime. ___ ___ ___ _____

   c. Attach proximal end of tubing to pump and distal end to epidural catheter. Tape all connections. Start infusion. ___ ___ ___ _____

   d. Check infusion pump for proper calibration and operation. ___ ___ ___ _____

6. If worn, remove and dispose of gloves. ___ ___ ___ _____

7. Explain that nurses will be monitoring response to the epidural analgesic. ___ ___ ___ _____

8. Use Completion Protocol. ___ ___ ___ _____

Evaluation

1. Evaluate every hour for 24 hours, then at least every 4 hours, changes in level of consciousness, pain, and vital signs. ___ ___ ___ _____

2. Ask client to rate pain intensity. ___ ___ ___ _____

3. Evaluate integrity of dressing. ___ ___ ___ _____

4. Ask client if headache is present. ___ ___ ___ _____

5. Evaluate catheter insertion site for inflammation or pruritus. ___ ___ ___ _____

6. Evaluate rate and depth of respirations. ___ ___ ___ _____

	S	U	NP	Comments
7. Assess sedation level, level of consciousness, and orientation.	___	___	___	_____
8. Monitor for voiding pattern and for bladder distention.	___	___	___	_____
9. Ask client if pruritus is present.	___	___	___	_____
• Identify unexpected outcomes and intervene as necessary.	___	___	___	_____
• Record and report intervention and client's response.	___	___	___	_____

Performance Checklist: Skill 11.5

Local Anesthetic Infusion Pump for Management of Postoperative Pain

	S	U	NP	Comments

Assessment

1. Perform complete pain assessment.

2. Inspect surgical dressing.

3. Observe label on device for type of anesthetic, strength, and infusion rate.

Implementation

1. Use Standard Protocol.

2. Review surgeon's note.

3. Assess surgical dressing and site of catheter insertion.
   a. Assess catheter connections.
   b. Assess for blood backing up tubing.
   c. Read label on device.

4. Determine extremity activity level from physician's orders.

5. Assess for signs of Marcaine toxicity.

6. For catheter removal order:
   a. Remove surgical dressing using clean gloves.
   b. Wash hands with soap and water for at least 2 minutes and then apply sterile gloves.
   c. Have client sit in relaxed position.
   d. Have client sit with leg up and supported if knee is surgical site.
   e. Encourage client to take a few deep breaths and relax.
   f. Grasp tube firmly and pull outward from skin with steady motion.
   g. Observe catheter tip for mark on end.
   h. Place catheter in plastic bag using standard precautions.
   i. Place a sterile dressing over the area and apply pressure for at least 2 minutes.
   j. Observe site for excessive bleeding or fluid loss. If none, apply an adherent dressing.

	S	U	NP	Comments

7. Document findings. ___ ___ ___ _____

8. Remind client of physician's follow-up
   appointment. ___ ___ ___ _____

9. Use Completion Protocol. ___ ___ ___ _____

Evaluation

1. Ask client to rate pain level. ___ ___ ___ _____

2. Evaluate PQRST aspects of pain. ___ ___ ___ _____

3. Observe client's position, mobility, relaxation,
   and ability to perform ADLs. ___ ___ ___ _____

4. Inspect condition of surgical dressing. ___ ___ ___ _____

- Identify unexpected outcomes and intervene as
  necessary. ___ ___ ___ _____

- Record and report intervention and client's
  response. ___ ___ ___ _____

Performance Checklist: Skill 12.1

Assessing Temperature, Pulse, Respirations, and Blood Pressure

	S	U	NP	Comments

Assessment

1. Identify daily fluctuations in vital signs. ____ ____ ____ _____

2. Identify medications or treatments that may influence vital signs. ____ ____ ____ _____

3. Identify factors that influence vital signs. ____ ____ ____ _____

4. Identify factors likely to interfere with the accuracy of vital sign measurement. ____ ____ ____ _____

5. Identify conditions that influence blood pressure. ____ ____ ____ _____

6. Identify pertinent related laboratory values. ____ ____ ____ _____

7. Determine baseline vital signs from client's record. ____ ____ ____ _____

8. Determine appropriate temperature site for client considering advantages and disadvantages of each site. ____ ____ ____ _____

9. Determine BP device most appropriate for client. ____ ____ ____ _____

Implementation

1. Use Standard Protocol. ____ ____ ____ _____

2. Assist client to comfortable position lying or sitting. ____ ____ ____ _____

3. Oral temperature
   a. Remove thermometer pack from charging unit and attach oral probe (blue) for oral or axillary or rectal (red) for rectal temperature. Grasp top of probe without pressure on ejection button. Press probe cover until locked in place. ____ ____ ____ _____
   b. Ask client to open mouth and place probe in posterior sublingual pocket. Have client close lips. ____ ____ ____ _____
   c. Leave thermometer in place until audible sound indicates completion and note reading. Remove from under tongue. Inform client of temperature reading, and record. ____ ____ ____ _____

d. Push ejection button on thermometer probe to discard probe cover. Return probe to storage position and thermometer to charger.

_____ _____ _____ _____

Nurse Alert: Repeat measurement if abnormal.

4. Tympanic temperature
   a. Assist client in assuming comfortable position with head turned toward side away from nurse.

_____ _____ _____ _____

   b. Remove thermometer handheld unit from charging base being careful not to apply pressure to the ejection button. Slide disposable speculum cover over otoscope-like tip until it locks in place. Do not touch lens cover.

_____ _____ _____ _____

   c. If holding unit with right hand, obtain reading from client's right ear (use left ear if left-handed).

_____ _____ _____ _____

   d. For an adult, pull the pinna back, up, and out. Note presence of cerumen.

_____ _____ _____ _____

   e. Pointing toward the nose, insert speculum into ear canal snugly to seal the canal from ambient air temperature. Refer to manufacturer's instructions for any additional specific directions.

_____ _____ _____ _____

   f. Upon placement, depress scan button on unit. Leave thermometer in place until audible signal occurs and temperature appears on display.

_____ _____ _____ _____

   g. Carefully remove speculum from auditory meatus. Push ejection button on thermometer stem to discard speculum cover.

_____ _____ _____ _____

   h. Inform client of temperature reading. Repeat measurement in other ear if temperature is abnormal, or wait and repeat in same ear after 2 to 3 minutes. Consider an alternative site.

_____ _____ _____ _____

   i. Return handheld unit to charger base.

_____ _____ _____ _____

5. Rectal temperature
   a. Apply gloves. Provide privacy. Assist client to Sims' position with upper leg flexed. Remove bed linens or clothes, exposing only anal area.

_____ _____ _____ _____

   b. Remove thermometer pack from charging unit and attach rectal probe (red) to unit. Slide disposable plastic probe cover over thermometer until it locks in place.

_____ _____ _____ _____

   c. Squeeze liberal amount of lubricant onto tissue. Dip thermometer probe end into lubricant, covering 1 to 1½ inches (2.5-3.5 cm) for adult.

_____ _____ _____ _____

	S	U	NP	Comments

d. With nondominant hand, separate client's buttocks to expose anus. Ask client to breathe slowly and relax. ___ ___ ___ _____

e. Gently insert thermometer into anus in direction of umbilicus, 1½ inches (3.5 cm) for adult. Do not force thermometer. Withdraw thermometer if resistance is felt. ___ ___ ___ _____

f. Hold thermometer probe in place until audible signal occurs and temperature appears on display. Remove thermometer probe from anus. ___ ___ ___ _____

g. Push ejection button on probe stem to discard plastic cover. Return thermometer stem to storage position on unit. ___ ___ ___ _____

h. Wipe client's anal area with soft tissue. Discard tissue and remove gloves. ___ ___ ___ _____

i. Inform client of temperature reading and record. Return thermometer to charger. ___ ___ ___ _____

6. Axillary temperature

a. Provide privacy. Assist client to supine or sitting position and move clothing or gown away from shoulder and arm. ___ ___ ___ _____

b. Remove thermometer pack from charging unit and attach oral (blue tip) probe to unit. Grasp top of probe stem and slide disposable plastic probe cover over thermometer stem until cover locks in place. ___ ___ ___ _____

c. Raise client's arm away from torso. Dry axilla if excess perspiration is present. Insert thermometer probe into center of axilla, lower arm over probe, and place arm across client's chest. ___ ___ ___ _____

Nurse Alert: In an infant or young child it may be necessary to hold the arm against the child's side.

d. Hold thermometer probe in place until audible signal occurs and temperature appears on display. Remove thermometer probe from axilla. Inform client of temperature reading and record. ___ ___ ___ _____

e. Push ejection button on probe stem to discard plastic cover. Return thermometer probe stem to storage position on unit. Return thermometer to charger. ___ ___ ___ _____

7. Pulse

a. Position client's forearm and slightly flex the wrist with palm down. ___ ___ ___ _____

b. Place tips of first two fingers of hand over groove along the radial or thumb side of the client's inner wrist. ___ ___ ___ _____

	S	U	NP	Comments

c. Lightly compress against radius, obliterate pulse initially, and then relax pressure so pulse becomes easily palpable.

d. Determine strength of pulse.

e. After pulse can be felt regularly, begin to count rate. If pulse is regular, count rate for 30 seconds and multiple total by 2. If pulse is irregular, count rate for 60 seconds. Assess frequency and pattern of irregularity.

Nurse Alert: Assess for pulse deficit using apical or radial pulse with colleague.

8. Respirations
   a. Without changing the position of your hand on the pulse, observe one complete respiratory cycle.
   b. After cycle is observed, look at watch's second hand and begin to count rate.
   c. If rhythm is regular, count number of respirations in 30 seconds and multiply by 2. If rhythm is irregular, less than 12 or greater than 20, count for 1 full minute.
   d. Note depth of respirations.
   e. Note rhythm of ventilatory cycle.
   f. Observe for evidence of increased effort to inhale and exhale.

Nurse Alert: Apnea or respiratory rate less than 12 or greater than 20 and hypoventilation may need immediate attention.

9. Manual auscultation of upper extremity blood pressure
   a. Determine the best site for BP assessment.
   b. Select appropriate cuff size.

Nurse Alert: Eliminate extraneous noise.

   c. Expose upper arm by removing restrictive clothing.
   d. With client sitting or lying, position client's forearm, supported with palm turned up at level of the heart.
   e. Palpate brachial artery.
   f. Position cuff 1 inch (2.5 cm) above site of brachial pulsation (antecubital space). Center bladder of cuff above artery. With cuff fully deflated, wrap cuff evenly and snugly around upper arm.
   g. Position manometer vertically at eye level. Observer should be no farther than 1 yard away.

h. Estimate systolic BP if baseline not known. Palpate the brachial or radial while inflating cuff rapidly to pressure 30 mm Hg above point at which pulse disappears. Slowly deflate cuff and note point when pulse reappears.

i. Deflate cuff fully and wait 30 seconds.

j. Place stethoscope earpieces in ears, and be sure sounds are clear.

k. Relocate brachial artery and place bell or diaphragm chest piece of stethoscope over it. Do not allow chest piece to touch cuff or clothing.

l. Close valve of pressure bulb clockwise until tight.

m. Rapidly inflate cuff to 30 mm Hg above palpated systolic pressure.

n. Slowly release pressure bulb valve and allow mercury (or needle of aneroid manometer gauge) to fall at rate of 2 to 3 mm Hg/second.

Nurse Alert: If you hear sounds immediately, start again after waiting 60 seconds.

o. Note point on manometer when first clear sound is heard.

p. Continue to deflate cuff gradually, noting point at which sound disappears in adults. Note pressure to nearest 2 mm Hg. Listen for 10 to 20 mm Hg after the last sound, and then allow remaining air to escape quickly.

q. If this is first assessment of client, repeat procedure on other arm.

r. Remove cuff from client's arm unless measurement must be repeated.

s. Record readings from both arms. Use arm with highest BP measurement for all subsequent BP recordings.

t. Inform client of the BP.

10. Use Completion Protocol.

Evaluation

1. Compare vital signs with client's baseline and expected ranges.

2. Evaluate client's understanding of factors that influence vital signs.

3. Identify baseline for clients with chronic diseases.

4. Ask client to describe changes in vital signs related to therapies.

	S	U	NP	Comments

- Identify unexpected outcomes and nursing interventions. ___ ___ ___ _____

- Record and report intervention and client's response. ___ ___ ___ _____

Performance Checklist: Procedural Guideline 12.1

Electronic Blood Pressure Measurement

		S	U	NP	Comments
1.	Use Standard Protocol.				
2.	Do not delegate this skill to assistive personnel.				
3.	Determine appropriateness of using electronic measurement.				
4.	Determine best site for cuff placement.				
5.	Assist client to comfortable position, lying or sitting. Place electronic BP machine near client and plug machine into source of electricity.				
6.	Locate on/off switch and turn machine on for self-test of system.				
7.	Select appropriate cuff size for extremity and machine.				
8.	Expose extremity by removing restrictive clothing.				
9.	Prepare BP cuff by squeezing all the air out and connecting cuff to connector hose.				
10.	Wrap cuff snugly around extremity, with "artery" marker correctly placed.				
11.	Verify that connector hose between cuff and machine is not kinked.				
12.	Set the frequency control for automatic or manual according to manufacturer's instructions, then press the start button.				
13.	Determine the frequency of measurement and client-specific alarm limits according to physician's order or nursing judgment. (Follow manufacturer's instructions.)				
14.	Leave the cuff in place if measurements will be frequent. Remove cuff at least every 2 hours to assess underlying skin integrity. Alternate sites, if possible.				
15.	Compare electronic readings with auscultatory BP as ordered, usually every 1 to 2 hours.				

16. Use the auscultatory method if electronic BP measurements are difficult to obtain or appear inaccurate.

____ ____ ____ _____

17. Use Completion Protocol.

____ ____ ____ _____

Performance Checklist: Skill 13.1

General Survey

	S	U	NP	Comments

Assessment

1. Note if client has experienced any acute distress.

Nurse Alert: Findings may change the direction of the examination.

2. Review graphic sheet for vital signs and consider factors that may influence findings.

3. Determine client's primary language. Obtain interpreter if necessary.

4. Reconfirm primary reason client has sought health care.

5. Identify client's normal height and weight. Determine whether client has been dieting or exercising.

6. Review client's past I&O.

7. Identify client's general perceptions about personal health.

8. Assess for evidence of latex allergy.

Implementation

1. Use Standard Protocol.

2. Explain procedure to client.

3. Note client's verbal and nonverbal behaviors. Determine level of consciousness and orientation.

4. Obtain vital signs.

5. Observe client's overall appearance.

6. Determine client's understanding of questions.

7. For inappropriate client responses, ask short, focused questions.

8. Offer simple commands if client is unable to respond to questions.

	S	U	NP	Comments

Nurse Alert: A more specialized assessment may be indicated if the client responds inappropriately. Marked changes in mental status should be reported immediately.

9.   Assess affect and mood.   ___ ___ ___ _____

10.   Observe client's interaction with others.   ___ ___ ___ _____

Nurse Alert: Be discreet in how interview is handled. It may be necessary to delay the assessment until significant other is not present.

11.   Assess posture.
   a. Observe body movements.   ___ ___ ___ _____
   b. Note if movements are coordinated.   ___ ___ ___ _____

12.   Assess speech.   ___ ___ ___ _____

13.   Observe hygiene and grooming.
   a. Observe condition of hair.   ___ ___ ___ _____
   b. Inspect condition of nails.   ___ ___ ___ _____
   c. Assess presence or absence of body odor.   ___ ___ ___ _____

14.   Assess the eyes.
   a. Inspect appearance and movement of eyes.   ___ ___ ___ _____
   b. Note near and far vision.   ___ ___ ___ _____
   c. Inspect pupils.   ___ ___ ___ _____
   d. Test pupillary reflexes with penlight.   ___ ___ ___ _____

15.   Assess hearing. Note response to questions and use of hearing aid.   ___ ___ ___ _____

Nurse Alert: If hearing deficit is present, inspect client's ears to determine presence of impacted cerumen, external otitis, or swelling in ear canal.

16.   Inspect nares on clients with nasal tubes.   ___ ___ ___ _____

17.   Assess the condition of the mouth: oral mucosa, tongue, teeth, and gums. Determine whether client wears dentures or retainers.   ___ ___ ___ _____

18.   Ask if client has noted changes in the skin.   ___ ___ ___ _____

19.   Inspect skin surfaces. Compare symmetrical body parts.   ___ ___ ___ _____

Nurse Alert: Be alert for basal cell carcinomas, often seen in sun-exposed areas.

20.   Carefully inspect color of face, oral mucosa, lips, conjunctivae, sclera, palms of hands, and nail beds.   ___ ___ ___ _____

Nurse Alert: For clients with bandages, casts, restraints, or other restrictive devices, note areas of pallor and decreased temperature. Immediate release of pressure from restrictive device may be necessary.

	S	U	NP	Comments

21. Use fingertips to palpate skin surfaces for texture and moisture.
   a. Using dorsum (back) of hand, palpate skin temperature, noting differences. ____ ____ ____ _____
   b. Assess skin turgor by grasping fold of skin on the sternum, forearm, or abdomen with the fingertips. Release skinfold and note ease and speed with which skin returns to place. ____ ____ ____ _____

22. Apply gloves. Inspect character of any secretions. ____ ____ ____ _____

23. Assess skin for presence of pressure areas. For areas of redness, place fingertip over area and apply gentle pressure, then release. ____ ____ ____ _____

Nurse Alert: Evidence of normal reactive hyperemia must result in repositioning the client and development of turning schedule.

24. Carefully inspect any lesions that are detected.
   a. Gently palpate lesion to determine mobility, contour, and consistency. Apply gloves if drainage is noted. ____ ____ ____ _____
   b. Note if client reports tenderness on palpation. ____ ____ ____ _____
   c. Measure size of lesion. ____ ____ ____ _____

25. Apply clean gloves and palpate IV site. Note when site is due to be changed. ____ ____ ____ _____

26. Check the IV fluids and medications, including type, rate, and expiration dates. ____ ____ ____ _____

27. Observe for signs of abuse for child, female, or older adult. ____ ____ ____ _____

Nurse Alert: A pattern of findings indicating abuse usually mandates a report. Consult immediately with the physician, social worker, and other support staff to facilitate placement of client in safer environment.

28. Use Completion Protocol. ____ ____ ____ _____

Evaluation

1. Observe throughout the assessment for evidence of distress. ____ ____ ____ _____

2. Compare assessment findings with previous observations. ____ ____ ____ _____

3. Ask the client if there is information about physical condition that has not been discussed. ____ ____ ____ _____

• Identify unexpected outcomes and intervene as necessary.

• Record and report intervention and client's response. ____ ____ ____ _____

Performance Checklist: Skill 13.3

Assessing the Heart and Neck Vessels

	S	U	NP	Comments

Assessment

1. Assess client for risk factors for heart or vascular disease. ___ ___ ___ _____

2. Determine whether client is taking medication for cardiovascular function. ___ ___ ___ _____

3. Ask if client has experienced signs or symptoms of cardiovascular or respiratory problems. ___ ___ ___ _____

4. Determine characteristics of chest pain. ___ ___ ___ _____

5. Assess family history of risk factors for heart disease. ___ ___ ___ _____

6. Ask client about personal history of cardiovascular disease. ___ ___ ___ _____

Implementation

1. Use Standard Protocol. ___ ___ ___ _____

2. Assist client to relax and be as comfortable as possible. ___ ___ ___ _____

3. Have client assume semi-Fowler's or supine position. ___ ___ ___ _____

4. Explain procedure. ___ ___ ___ _____

5. Ensure that room is quiet. ___ ___ ___ _____

6. Form an image of the location of the heart in your mind. ___ ___ ___ _____

7. Find the angle of Louis, which is felt as a ridge in the sternum approximately 2 inches (5 cm) below the sternal notch. ___ ___ ___ _____

8. Find the following anatomical landmarks:
   a. The 2nd intercostal space on the right is the aortic area. ___ ___ ___ _____
   b. The 2nd intercostal space on the left is the pulmonic area. ___ ___ ___ _____
   c. Erb's point (2nd pulmonic area) is at the 3rd intercostal space. ___ ___ ___ _____
   d. The tricuspid area is at the 4th intercostal space. ___ ___ ___ _____

e. The mitral area is located at the 5th intercostal space at the left midclavicular line.

___ ___ ___ _____

f. The epigastric area is at tip of the sternum.

___ ___ ___ _____

9. Stand to client's right and look first at precordium with client supine. Note any visible pulsations or lifts.

___ ___ ___ _____

Nurse Alert: Presence of a thrill is not normal and may indicate a disruption of blood flow.

10. Locate the PMI by palpating along the 5th intercostal space in the midclavicular line.

___ ___ ___ _____

11. If palpating the PMI is difficult, turn client onto left side.

___ ___ ___ _____

Nurse Alert: A stronger than expected impulse may be a heave or a lift.

12. Inspect the epigastric area and palpate the abdominal aorta.

___ ___ ___ _____

13. Auscultate heart sounds with client sitting, supine, and in left lateral recumbent position.

___ ___ ___ _____

14. Ask client not to speak. Place stethoscope's diaphragm lightly against chest wall, then alternate with bell.

a. Listen at the apex or PMI then move to tricuspid, pulmonic, and aortic areas.

___ ___ ___ _____

b. Listen for S_2 at each site.

___ ___ ___ _____

c. After both sounds are heard clearly as "lub-dub," count each combination of S_1 and S_2 as one heartbeat for 1 minute.

___ ___ ___ _____

d. Assess heart rhythm.

___ ___ ___ _____

e. When heart rate is irregular, compare apical and radial pulses.

___ ___ ___ _____

15. Continue to auscultate for extra heart sounds. Note characteristics of abnormal sounds.

a. Listen for gallops and rubs.

___ ___ ___ _____

b. Listen for clicks.

___ ___ ___ _____

c. Listen for friction rubs.

___ ___ ___ _____

16. Auscultate for heart murmurs.

___ ___ ___ _____

17. Note where murmur, if present, is best heard.

___ ___ ___ _____

18. Note pitch of murmur.

___ ___ ___ _____

19. Assess carotid arteries with client in sitting position.

___ ___ ___ _____

20. Inspect neck bilaterally for obvious pulsations.

___ ___ ___ _____

	S	U	NP	Comments

21. Palpate each artery separately with index and middle fingers. Note if pulsation changes with inspiration or expiration.

Nurse Alert: Do not vigorously palpate or massage the arteries.

22. Place bell of stethoscope over each carotid artery, auscultating for blowing sound or bruit.

23. Assess jugular veins with client in 45- to 90-degree position. Check for visible pulsation.

Nurse Alert: Visible jugular pulsation suggests immediate treatment.

24. Use Completion Protocol.

Evaluation

1. Compare findings with client's baseline and expected findings.

2. Ask another nurse to confirm assessment if heart sounds or pulses are not audible or palpable.

3. Determine client's understanding of risk factors and health promotion measures.

- Identify unexpected outcomes and intervene as necessary.

- Record and report intervention and client's response.

Name _____ Date _____ Instructor's Name _____

Performance Checklist: Skill 13.4

Assessing the Abdomen

	S	U	NP	Comments

Assessment

1. Elicit details of abdominal or low back pain. _____ _____ _____ _____

2. Note position and movement of client. _____ _____ _____ _____

3. Obtain detailed data about elimination patterns for bowel and bladder along with measures used to promote elimination. _____ _____ _____ _____

4. Inquire about history of abdominal or GI surgeries. _____ _____ _____ _____

5. Determine whether client has had nausea, vomiting, or cramping within the past 24 hours. _____ _____ _____ _____

6. Assess for GI signs and symptoms. _____ _____ _____ _____

7. Determine whether client takes antiinflammatory medication or antibiotics. _____ _____ _____ _____

8. Assess family history of cancer, kidney disease, alcoholism, drug use, and hypertension. _____ _____ _____ _____

9. For female clients, determine whether they are pregnant. _____ _____ _____ _____

10. Review history for possible occupational exposures. _____ _____ _____ _____

Implementation

1. Use Standard Protocol. _____ _____ _____ _____

2. Prepare client.
   a. Ask if client needs to urinate or defecate. _____ _____ _____ _____
   b. Keep upper chest and legs draped. _____ _____ _____ _____
   c. Be sure that room is warm. _____ _____ _____ _____
   d. Expose area from just above xiphoid to symphysis pubis. _____ _____ _____ _____
   e. Have client assume supine or recumbent position with knees slightly flexed or a small pillow under knees. _____ _____ _____ _____
   f. Maintain conversation during assessment. Explain steps calmly and slowly. _____ _____ _____ _____
   g. Ask client to point to tender areas. _____ _____ _____ _____

Nurse Alert: Observe respirations as position is changed.

	S	U	NP	Comments

3. Identify landmarks that divide abdominal region into quadrants.

4. Inspect abdominal surface for skin alterations.

5. Ask if client self-administers medication if bruising is noted.

Nurse Alert: Bruising may indicate physical abuse, accidental injury, or bleeding disorders.

6. Inspect for contour and symmetry. Note any masses, bulging, or distention.

7. If abdomen appears distended, note if it is generalized and extends to the flanks.

8. If distention is suspected, measure size of abdominal girth by placing tape measure around abdomen at level of umbilicus and note measurement. Mark site with marker pen.

9. If nasogastric or intestinal tubes are present and connected to suction, turn off momentarily.

10. Auscultate abdomen by placing diaphragm of stethoscope lightly over each of the four quadrants. Ask client not to speak. Listen 2 to 5 minutes for succession of clicks or gurgles in each quadrant before deciding bowel sounds are absent.

Nurse Alert: Severe paralytic ileus may be accompanied by nausea, vomiting, increasing distention, and inability to pass flatus.

11. Place the bell of the stethoscope over the epigastric region and auscultate vascular sounds.

Nurse Alert: Note the presence of an aortic bruit and notify the physician immediately. Do not palpate over an abdominal bruit.

12. With client supine, gently percuss each of the four quadrants of the abdomen. Note areas of tympany and dullness.

13. Ask client if abdomen feels unusually tight, and determine when this developed.

14. With client sitting, gently but firmly percuss over each costovertebral angle along the scapular lines. Use ulnar surface of fist to percuss directly against the client's skin or indirectly by placing the nondominant hand flat against the costovertebral angle and percussing with the dominant hand. Note if client experiences pain.

	S	U	NP	Comments

15. Lightly palpate over abdominal quadrants. Keep the palm and forearm horizontal. The pads of the fingertips depress the skin approximately 1/2 inch (1 cm). _____ _____ _____ _____

Nurse Alert: Palpate painful areas last. Avoid quick jabs.

    a. Note muscle tone, abdominal stiffness, presence of masses, and tenderness. Observe client's face for grimacing, which may indicate tenderness or pain. _____ _____ _____ _____

    b. Note if abdomen is firm or soft to touch. _____ _____ _____ _____

16. Palpate for a smooth, rounded mass just below the umbilicus and above the symphysis pubis. Ask if client has the sensation to void. _____ _____ _____ _____

Nurse Alert: Routinely check for distended bladder if client is unable to void, is incontinent, or has an indwelling catheter that is not draining well.

17. If abdominal masses are palpated, note size, location, shape, consistency, tenderness, mobility, and texture. _____ _____ _____ _____

18. If tenderness is present, check for rebound tenderness. _____ _____ _____ _____

19. Perform deep palpation, being sure that the client is relaxed. Depress the palm and fingers approximately 1 to 3 inches (2.5-7.5 cm) into the abdomen. _____ _____ _____ _____

20. Use Completion Protocol. _____ _____ _____ _____

Evaluation

1. Observe throughout the assessment for evidence of discomfort. _____ _____ _____ _____

2. Compare findings with client's baseline and expected findings. _____ _____ _____ _____

• Identify unexpected outcomes and intervene as necessary. _____ _____ _____ _____

• Record and report intervention and client's response. _____ _____ _____ _____

Performance Checklist: Skill 13.5

Assessing the Extremities and Peripheral Circulation

	S	U	NP	Comments

Assessment

1. Review client's history for risk of osteoporosis. _____ _____ _____ _____

2. Ask client to describe history of alteration of bone, muscle, or joint function, and location of alteration. _____ _____ _____ _____

3. Assess nature and extent of client's pain. _____ _____ _____ _____

4. Determine how client's alteration influences ADLs and social function. _____ _____ _____ _____

5. Assess height decrease in women over 50 years of age. _____ _____ _____ _____

6. Ask whether client experiences cardiovascular signs and symptoms, such as dyspnea, chest pain, excess fatigue. _____ _____ _____ _____

7. Ask whether client experiences cramps, numbness or tingling, sensation of cold, or swelling of the extremities. _____ _____ _____ _____

Implementation

1. Use Standard Protocol. _____ _____ _____ _____

2. Prepare client.
   a. Integrate musculoskeletal assessment during other parts of the physical assessment or during nursing care. _____ _____ _____ _____
   b. Plan time for rest periods during assessment. _____ _____ _____ _____

3. Observe ability to use arms and hands for grasping objects. _____ _____ _____ _____

4. Assess muscle strength of upper extremities. _____ _____ _____ _____

5. To assess hand grasp strength, ask client to grasp the fingers of both hands and squeeze. Note weakness, and compare right with left. _____ _____ _____ _____

6. Have client resist pressure applied by moving against the resistance. Compare the right and left sides. _____ _____ _____ _____

7. If muscle weakness is identified, measure muscle size with a tape measure. Compare both sides. _____ _____ _____ _____

	S	U	NP	Comments

8. Observe position for supine, prone, sitting, and standing.

9. Inspect gait as client stands and walks.

10. Stand behind client and observe postural alignment. Look sideways at cervical, thoracic, and lumbar curves.

11. Make a general observation of the extremities, checking overall size, alignment, and symmetry.

12. Gently palpate bones, joints, and surrounding tissue. Note any inflammation, tenderness, or resistance to pressure.

13. Ask client to put joints through full range of motion (ROM). Observe equality of motion from side to side.
    a. Active motion: Instruct client in moving each joint through normal ROM. Demonstration may be necessary.
    b. Passive motion: Have client relax and move the same joints passively, supporting extremities at the joints.

14. Palpate joints for presence of inflammation and tenderness.

15. Assess muscle tone in major muscle groups.

16. Inspect lower extremities for changes in color and condition of the skin. Note skin and nail texture, hair distribution, venous patterns, edema, and scars or ulcers. Compare skin color lying and standing.

17. Palpate edematous areas, noting mobility, consistency, and tenderness.

18. Assess for pitting edema by pressing area firmly for 5 seconds, then releasing.

19. Check capillary refill and note color of nail bed.

20. Ask if client has tenderness or pain in legs, then palpate for heat, firmness, or localized swelling of the calf muscle.

Nurse Alert: Homans' sign is no longer a reliable indicator for the presence of deep vein thrombosis (DVT).

21. Palpate each peripheral artery, starting at most distal part of each extremity, for elasticity of vessel wall: Depressing and releasing artery, note ease with which it springs back to shape. Note strength and rhythm of pulse.

22. Palpate radial pulse at groove along radial side of forearm, lateral to flexor tendon of wrist.

___ ___ ___ _____

23. Palpate ulnar pulse along ulnar side of forearm.

___ ___ ___ _____

24. Palpate brachial pulse at groove between biceps and triceps muscles above elbow at antecubital fossa.

___ ___ ___ _____

25. Have client lie supine with feet relaxed and palpate dorsalis pedis between great and first toe, moving fingers along groove between extensor tendons until pulse is palpable.

___ ___ ___ _____

26. If the pedal pulses are difficult to palpate or not palpable, use a Doppler instrument over pulse site.

___ ___ ___ _____

   a. Apply conducting gel to the client's skin over the pulse site or onto the transducer tip of probe.

___ ___ ___ _____

   b. Turn Doppler on. Gently apply probe to skin, changing angle until pulsation is audible. Adjust volume as needed.

___ ___ ___ _____

27. Palpate posterior tibial pulse by having client relax and slightly extend feet. Place fingertips behind and below medial malleolus.

___ ___ ___ _____

28. Palpate popliteal pulse by having client slightly flex knee with foot resting on table or bed. Instruct client to keep leg muscles relaxed. Palpate deeply into popliteal fossa with fingers of both hands placed just lateral to midline. Client may also lie prone.

___ ___ ___ _____

29. Palpate femoral pulse with client supine by placing first two fingers over inguinal area below inguinal ligament and midway between pubic symphysis and anterosuperior iliac spine.

___ ___ ___ _____

30. Monitor deep tendon reflexes for clients with back pain or surgery, CVA, or spinal cord injury.

___ ___ ___ _____

31. Test deep tendon reflexes, if indicated.
   a. Knee reflex. Palpate the patellar tendon just below the patella. Tap the pointed end of the reflex hammer briskly on the tendon.

___ ___ ___ _____

   b. Plantar response (Babinski's reflex). Using the handle end of the reflex hammer, stroke the lateral aspect of the sole from the heel to the ball of the foot.

___ ___ ___ _____

	S	U	NP	Comments

32. Use Completion Protocol.   ___ ___ ___ _____

Evaluation

1. Compare muscle strength and ROM with previous shift assessment.   ___ ___ ___ _____

2. Compare pulses and capillary refill bilaterally with previous shift assessment.   ___ ___ ___ _____

3. Compare absence or presence and extent of edema with previous shift assessment.   ___ ___ ___ _____

4. Evaluate level of client's discomfort after procedure.   ___ ___ ___ _____

- Identify unexpected outcomes and intervene as necessary.   ___ ___ ___ _____

- Record and report intervention and client's response.   ___ ___ ___ _____

Performance Checklist: Skill 14.1

Urine Specimen Collection—Mid-Stream, Sterile Urinary Catheter

	S	U	NP	Comments

Assessment

1. Assess client's ability to assist with specimen collection.

2. Assess client's understanding of need for specimen.

3. Determine whether fluid, dietary requirements, or medications need to be administered along with the test.

4. Assess for signs and symptoms of urinary tract infection.

5. Assess urinary elimination pattern.

Implementation

1. Use Standard Protocol.

2. Explain to client and family member reason for specimen collection, how client can assist, and how to obtain specimen.

3. Collect clean voided urine specimen.
   a. Give client or family member towel, washcloth, and soap to cleanse perineum, or assist client (Apply gloves). Bedridden client may be positioned on bedpan.
   b. Using sterile technique, open commercial specimen kit.
   c. Open specimen container and place cap with sterile inside and surface up. Do not touch inside of container.
   d. Have client cleanse perineum and collect specimen independently, if possible. Review proper cleansing of perineum. Provide assistance, if necessary.
      (1) Male: Hold penis with one hand and, using circular motion and antiseptic towelette, cleanse from meatus outward in a circular motion. Retract the foreskin of uncircumcised males.
      (2) Female: Spread labia minora with fingers of nondominant hand. Use

       dominant hand to cleanse with
       antiseptic towelette, moving from
       front to back in single strokes.   ——— ——— ————————————

   e. Rinse area with sterile water and dry with
      cotton. Refer to agency policy.   ——— ——— ————————————

   f. While holding foreskin or separating labia,
     have client initiate urine stream.   ——— ——— ————————————

   g. After urinary stream is achieved, pass
      specimen container into stream and
      collect 30 to 60 ml of urine.   ——— ——— ————————————

   h. Remove specimen container before flow
      of urine stops and before releasing
      foreskin or labia. Client should finish
      voiding in bedpan or toilet.   ——— ——— ————————————

   i. Replace cap securely on specimen
     container, touching only the outside.   ——— ——— ————————————

   j. Cleanse urine from exterior surface of
     container.   ——— ——— ————————————

Nurse Alert: Indicate on the laboratory slip if the client is menstruating.

4.   Collect urine from an indwelling urinary
    catheter.

   a. Explain that the procedure will cause no
     discomfort.   ——— ——— ————————————

   b. Explain why the catheter will be clamped
     for 30 minutes.   ——— ——— ————————————

   c. Clamp drainage tubing with clamp or
     rubber band for up to 30 minutes below
     the site of withdrawal.   ——— ——— ————————————

   d. Apply gloves. Position the catheter and
     cleanse entry port or self-sealing
     diaphragm with disinfectant swab.   ——— ——— ————————————

   e. Insert needle of syringe at 90-degree angle
     through entry port or at a 30-degree angle
     for self-sealing diaphragm and withdraw
     necessary volume of urine (3 ml for
     culture, 20 ml for routine urinalysis).   ——— ——— ————————————

   f. Transfer urine from syringe to appropriate
     container, depending on type of test to be
     done.   ——— ——— ————————————

   g. Do not recap needle. Dispose of needle
     in appropriate sharps receptacle.   ——— ——— ————————————

   h. Place lid tightly on specimen container.   ——— ——— ————————————

   i. Unclamp catheter and allow urine to flow
     into drainage bag. Observe that urine
     flows freely.   ——— ——— ————————————

5.   Securely attach properly completed
    identification label and laboratory requisition
    to the side of the specimen container.   ——— ——— ————————————

6.   Send specimen and requisition to laboratory
    as soon as possible, no longer than 2 hours.   ——— ——— ————————————

	S	U	NP	Comments

7. Use Completion Protocol. _____ _____ _____ _____

Evaluation

1. Ask client to identify steps in specimen collection procedure. _____ _____ _____ _____

2. Ask client to state purposes of specimen collection. _____ _____ _____ _____

3. Inspect clean voided specimen for contamination. _____ _____ _____ _____

- Identify unexpected outcomes and intervene as necessary. _____ _____ _____ _____

- Record and report intervention and client's response. _____ _____ _____ _____

Performance Checklist: Procedural Guideline 14.1

Collecting 24-Hour Timed Specimens

	S	U	NP	Comments

Implementation

1. Use Standard Protocol. _____ _____ _____ _____

2. Explain to client or family member reason for specimen collection, how client can assist, and how to obtain specimen. _____ _____ _____ _____

3. Have client drink two to four glasses of water about 30 minutes before timed collection. _____ _____ _____ _____

4. Apply gloves. Discard first specimen. Print time that test began on laboratory requisition. _____ _____ _____ _____

5. Place signs indicating timed urine specimen collection on client's door and toileting area. _____ _____ _____ _____

6. Measure volume of each voiding if I&O is being recorded. _____ _____ _____ _____

7. Place all voided urine in labeled specimen bottle with appropriate additive. _____ _____ _____ _____

Nurse Alert: It is essential for all urine to be collected for accurate test results. Timed collection must be restarted if urine is accidentally discarded or contaminated.

8. Keep specimen bottle in specimen refrigerator or container of ice in bathroom, unless otherwise instructed. _____ _____ _____ _____

9. Encourage client to drink two glasses of water 1 hour before the timed collection ends. _____ _____ _____ _____

10. Encourage client to empty bladder during last 14 minutes of timed collection period. _____ _____ _____ _____

11. Observe or ask whether urine has been saved throughout the collection period. _____ _____ _____ _____

12. Remove signs and inform client when collection period is completed. _____ _____ _____ _____

13. Attach completed identification label to side of specimen container and send container to laboratory as soon as possible. _____ _____ _____ _____

14. Use Completion Protocol. _____ _____ _____ _____

Performance Checklist: Procedural Guideline 14-2

Urine Screening for Glucose, Ketones, Protein, Blood, and pH

	S	U	NP	Comments

Implementation

1. Use Standard Protocol.

2. Ask client to collect a fresh random urine specimen. If client is catheterized, obtain a 5 ml specimen.

3. Apply gloves. Immerse end of chemically impregnated test strip into urine. Remove the strip immediately and tap it gently against the side of the collection container to remove excess urine.

4. Hold strip in horizontal position.

5. Precisely time the number of seconds specified on strip container, then compare the color of the test strip with the color chart.

6. Remove and discard gloves.

7. Discuss test results with client.

8. Use Completion Protocol.

Performance Checklist: Skill 14.2

Testing for Gastrointestinal Alterations (Stool Specimen, Hemoccult Test, Gastroccult Test)

	S	U	NP	Comments

Assessment

1. Assess client's medical history for GI disorders.

2. Assess female client's menstrual cycle.

3. Review medications for drugs that may cause GI bleeding.

4. Check physician's order for dietary restrictions before testing.

Implementation

1. Use Standard Protocol.

2. Discuss reason for specimen, how client can assist, and procedure for obtaining specimen.

3. Obtaining stool specimen:
   a. Assist client into bathroom or onto commode or bedpan. Instruct client to void and discard urine before defecating. Provide client clean, dry bedpan or specimen hat for defecation.
   b. Assist client in washing after toileting, if necessary. Return client to safe, comfortable position.
   c. Apply gloves. Take covered bedpan or container to bathroom or utility room and gather specimen:
      (1) Culture: Remove swab from sterile test tube, gather bean-sized piece of stool, and return swab to tube. Soak swab in liquid stool and return to tube.
      (2) Timed stool specimen: Place all of each stool in waxed cardboard containers for specific time ordered and keep in specimen refrigerator.
      (3) All other tests, including guaiac: Obtain specimen by using tongue blade to transfer portion of stool to container: 1 inch (2.5 cm) formed or 15 ml liquid stool.

    d. For timed test, place signs that read
       "Save all stool" over client's bed, on
       bathroom door, and above toilet.
    e. After obtaining specimen, place lid
       tightly on container.

4. Perform Hemoccult test.
    a. Use tip of wooden applicator to obtain
       small portion of feces.
    b. Open flap of Hemoccult slide and apply
       thin smear of stool on paper in the first
       box.
    c. Using the other end of the wooden
       applicator, obtain a second specimen
       from a different portion of the stool and
       apply thinly to slide's second box.
    d. Close slide cover and turn slide over to
       reverse side. Open cardboard flap and
       apply two drops of Hemoccult developing
       solution on each box of guaiac paper.
    e. Read results of test after 30 to 60 seconds,
       noting color changes.

5. Perform Gastroccult test
    a. To obtain specimen of gastric contents
       using nasogastric or nasoenteral tube,
       position client in high Fowler's position
       in bed or chair.
    b. Verify tube placement.
    c. Apply gloves. Collect gastric contents.
       Disconnect tube from suction or gravity
       drainage. Attach bulb or cone-tipped
       syringe. Aspirate 5 to 10 ml. Use a 3 ml
       syringe to obtain an emesis sample.
    d. Apply one drop of gastric sample to
       Gastroccult blood test slide using
       applicator or syringe.
    e. Apply two drops of commercial developer
       solution over sample and one drop
       between the positive and negative
       performance monitors on the slide.
    f. After 60 seconds, compare the color of
       the gastric sample with the performance
       monitors.
    g. Verify that the performance monitor
       turns blue in 30 seconds, indicating slide
       is working properly.

6. Explain test results to client.

7. Dispose of test slide, wooden applicator, and
    1 ml syringe in proper receptacle.

8. Reconnect nasogastric tube to drainage
    system, suction, or clamp, as ordered.

	S	U	NP	Comments

9. Remove and discard gloves.

10. Use Completion Protocol.

Evaluation

1. Observe characteristics of stool, emesis, or gastric secretions.

2. Compare test findings with expected results.

3. Ask client to explain the purpose of the test.

- Identify unexpected outcomes and intervene as necessary.

- Record and report intervention and client's response.

Performance Checklist: Skill 14.3

Blood Glucose Monitoring

	S	U	NP	Comments

Assessment

1. Assess client's understanding of procedure and purpose and importance of glucose monitoring.

2. Assess client for types of medications received.

3. Determine whether client has a low platelet count, is receiving anticoagulants, or has a bleeding disorder.

4. Determine whether specific conditions need to be met before or after sample collection.

5. Assess area of skin to be used as puncture site.

6. Review physician's order for frequency of measurement.

7. Assess client's ability to perform testing.

8. Assess client for signs and symptoms of glucose alterations.

9. Check the calibration of the equipment for accuracy.

Implementation

1. Use Standard Protocol.

2. Instruct client to wash hands with soap and warm water.

3. Position client comfortably in chair with hand lower than the heart.

4. Remove reagent strip from container and tightly reseal cap. Check expiration date.

5. Turn on glucose meter.

6. Insert strip into glucose meter and make adjustments as needed.

7. Remove reagent strip from meter and place on clean, dry surface with test pad facing up. Avoid touching reagent materials.

	S	U	NP	Comments

8. Apply gloves. Select a vascular area as a puncture site.

9. If finger is used, hold finger in dependent position while gently massaging toward the site.

10. Cleanse site with warm water or alcohol and allow to dry completely.

11. Remove cover of lancet or other device.

12. Place bloodletting device firmly against side of finger and push release button for needle to pierce the skin or hold the lancet perpendicular to the site and pierce finger quickly in one motion.

13. Wipe away the first droplet of blood with cotton ball. (Check the manufacturer's instructions for meter.)

14. Lightly squeeze puncture site until large droplet of blood has formed.

15. Hold reagent strip test pad close to drop of blood and transfer droplet to the test pad without smearing.

Nurse Alert: Repuncturing may be necessary if a large enough droplet is not formed.

16. Immediately press timer on meter and place reagent strip on towel on side of timer. Some meters require that the test strip be in the meter when the droplet of blood is applied.

17. Apply pressure to puncture site for at least 10 seconds. Check for continued bleeding. Continue to apply pressure as necessary.

18. When timer displays 60 seconds or sounds, use moderate pressure to wipe the blood from the test pad with a dry cotton ball.

19. While timer continues to count, place reagent strip into meter.

20. Read results on meter display.

21. Turn meter off.

22. Dispose of test strip, cotton balls, and lancet/bloodletting device appropriately.

23. Remove and discard gloves.

24. Share test results with client and encourage questions.

25. Use Completion Protocol.

	S	U	NP	Comments

Evaluation

1. Observe puncture site for evidence of bleeding or bruising. ___ ___ ___ _____

2. Compare glucose meter reading with expected blood glucose levels. ___ ___ ___ _____

3. Ask client to discuss procedure and test results. ___ ___ ___ _____

4. Observe client perform self-testing. ___ ___ ___ _____

• Identify unexpected outcomes and intervene as necessary. ___ ___ ___ _____

• Record and report intervention and client's response. ___ ___ ___ _____

Performance Checklist: Skill 14.4

Collecting Blood Specimens—Venipuncture with Vacutainer; Blood Cultures

	S	U	NP	Comments

Assessment

1. Assess if special conditions need to be met before specimen collection.

2. Assess client for possible risks of venipuncture (bleeding tendency, AV shunt, anticoagulant therapy).

3. Assess for contraindicated sites.

4. Review physician's order for type of tests.

5. Determine client's understanding of tests and ability to cooperate with procedure.

6. Assess for systemic evidence of bacteremia, if drawing specimen for blood culture.

Implementation

1. Use Standard Protocol.

2. Assist client to sit, lie supine or in semi-Fowler's position with arms supported and extended to form straight line from shoulders to wrists. Place small pillow or towel under upper arm.

3. Explain procedure to client.

4. Inspect extremity for best venipuncture site.

5. Apply gloves. Apply tourniquet (antecubital fossa site is most often used), making sure that it can be removed with a single motion.
   a. Position tourniquet 3 to 4 inches (5-10 cm) above venipuncture site selected.
   b. Cross tourniquet over client's arm, holding between fingers close to arm.
   c. Tuck loop between client's arm and tourniquet.
   d. Free end can be pulled to release tourniquet.

6. Palpate distal pulse below tourniquet. Reapply tourniquet if pulse not palpable.

Nurse Alert: It is recommended not to apply tourniquet on an older adult with poor skin turgor and fragile veins.

	S	U	NP	Comments

7. Keep tourniquet in place no longer than 1 minute.

8. Apply warm, wet compress over extremity for 10 minutes if unable to visualize or palpate vein.

9. Ask client to open and close fist several times, finally leaving fist clenched.

10. Palpate selected vein with fingers.

Nurse Alert: Do not vigorously tap or slap veins.

11. Obtain blood sample.
    a. Vacutainer specimen
       (1) Attach double-ended needle to vacuum tube.
       (2) Have proper blood specimen tube resting inside vacuum tube, but do not puncture rubber stopper.
       (3) Apply gloves. Cleanse venipuncture site with alcohol swab, moving in circular motion out from site for approximately 2 inches (5 cm). Allow to dry.
       (4) Remove needle cover and inform client that "stick" lasting only a few seconds will be felt. Client has better control over anxiety when prepared for what to expect.
       (5) Place thumb or forefinger of nondominant hand 1 inch (2.5 cm) above or below site and pull skin taut. Stretch skin down until vein is stabilized.
       (6) Hold vacuum tube at 15- to 30-degree angle from arm with bevel up.
       (7) Slowly insert needle into vein.
       (8) Grasp vacuum tube securely and advance specimen tube into needle of holder (do not advance needle in vein).
       (9) Note flow of blood into tube.
       (10) After specimen tube is filled, grasp vacuum tube firmly and remove tube. Insert additional specimen tubes. Insert additional specimen tubes as needed.

Nurse Alert: When filling tubes with anticoagulant additive, let tube fill until vacuum is exhausted. Rotate tube back and forth 8 to 10 times.

       (11) After last tube is filled, release tourniquet.

	S	U	NP	Comments

b. Blood culture
  (1) Carefully prepare proposed site with povidone-iodine (Betadine). Allow skin to dry.

  (2) Clean tops of the Vacutainer tubes or culture bottles with appropriate antiseptic.

  (3) Collect 10 to 15 ml of venous blood by venipuncture in a 20 ml syringe from each site.

  (4) Discard needle on syringe; replace with second sterile needle before injecting blood sample into culture bottle.

  (5) Place sample into anaerobic bottle first if both anaerobic and aerobic cultures are obtained.

  (6) Mix medium gently after inoculation.

12. Apply 2 × 2 gauze pad over puncture site without applying pressure and quickly but carefully withdraw needle from vein.

13. Immediately apply pressure over venipuncture site with gauze or antiseptic pad for 2 to 3 minutes or until bleeding stops. Inspect for bleeding at site and tape gauze dressing securely.

14. Take blood tubes containing additives; gently rotate back and forth 8 to 10 times.

15. Check tubes for any sign of external contamination with blood and decontaminate with 70% alcohol if necessary.

16. Dispose of needles, syringe, Vacutainer holder, and soiled equipment in proper container. Do not cap needles.

17. Remove disposable gloves after specimen is obtained and any spillage is cleaned.

18. Securely attach properly completed identification label to each tube and affix proper requisition.

19. Send specimens immediately to laboratory.

20. See Completion Protocol.

Evaluation

1. Ask client to explain purpose of tests.

2. Evaluate condition of venipuncture site.

3. Determine client's anxiety level.

4. Monitor laboratory test results.   _____ _____ _____ _____

• Identify unexpected outcomes and intervene as necessary.   _____ _____ _____ _____

• Record and report intervention and client's response.   _____ _____ _____ _____

Name _____ Date _____ Instructor's Name _____

Performance Checklist: Procedural Guideline 14-3

Venipuncture with Syringe

		S	U	NP	Comments
1.	Use Standard Protocol.				
2.	Apply gloves. Prepare for venipuncture (refer to Skill 14.4).				
3.	Have syringe with appropriate needle securely attached.				
4.	Cleanse venipuncture site with alcohol swab, moving in circular motion from site for approximately 2 inches (5 cm). Allow to dry.				
5.	Remove needle cover and inform client that "stick" lasting only a few seconds will be felt.				
6.	Place thumb or forefinger of nondominant hand 1 inch (2.5 cm) below site, and pull skin taut.				
7.	Hold syringe and needle at 15- to 30-degree angle from client's arm with bevel up.				
8.	Slowly insert needle into vein.				
9.	Hold syringe securely and pull back gently on plunger.				
10.	Obtain desired amount of blood, keeping needle stabilized.				
11.	After specimen is obtained, release tourniquet.				
12.	Continue with steps 13 through 19 in Skill 14.4.				
13.	Use Completion Protocol.				

Name _____ Date _____ Instructor's Name _____

Performance Checklist: Skill 14.5

Collecting Specimens from the Nose and Throat

	S	U	NP	Comments

Assessment

1. Assess condition of and drainage from nasal mucosa and sinuses.   ___ ___ ___ _____

2. Determine whether client has experienced postnasal drip, sinus headache or tenderness, nasal congestion, or sore throat.   ___ ___ ___ _____

3. Assess condition of posterior pharynx.   ___ ___ ___ _____

4. Assess for systemic indications of infection.   ___ ___ ___ _____

Implementation

1. Use Standard Protocol.   ___ ___ ___ _____

2. Ask client to sit erect in bed or chair facing you for nose or throat culture. Acutely ill client may lie back against bed with head of bed raised to 45-degree angle.   ___ ___ ___ _____

3. Have swab in tube ready for use.   ___ ___ ___ _____

4. Collect specimen
   a. Throat culture:
   (1) Apply gloves. Instruct client to tilt head backward. For clients in bed, place pillow behind shoulders.
   (2) Ask client to open mouth and say "ah."   ___ ___ ___ _____
   (3) If pharynx is not visualized, depress tongue with tongue blade and note inflamed areas of pharynx or tonsils. Depress anterior third of tongue only. (Illuminate with penlight as needed.)   ___ ___ ___ _____
   (4) Insert swab without touching lips, teeth, tongue, or cheeks.   ___ ___ ___ _____
   (5) Gently but quickly swab tonsillar area side to side, making contact with inflamed or purulent sites.   ___ ___ ___ _____
   b. Nasal culture:
   (1) Ask client to blow nose, and check nostrils for patency with penlight.   ___ ___ ___ _____
   (2) Ask client to tilt head back. Clients in bed should have pillow behind shoulders.   ___ ___ ___ _____

	S	U	NP	Comments

(3) Gently insert nasal speculum in one nostril (optional). Carefully pass swab through center of speculum (if used) into nostril until it reaches that portion of mucosa that is inflamed or containing. Rotate swab quickly.

(4) Remove swab without touching sides of speculum or nasal canal.

(5) Carefully remove nasal speculum (if used) and place in basin. Offer client facial tissue.

5. Immediately place swab in culture tube.

6. Cover end of tube with 2 × 2 gauze then crush ampule at bottom of tube, and push tip of swab into liquid medium.

7. Place top securely onto tube.

8. Discard supplies appropriately.

9. Attach ID label and requisition.

10. Enclose in plastic bag.

11. Send to laboratory immediately or refrigerate.

12. Remove and discard gloves.

13. Use Completion Protocol.

Evaluation

1. Ask client to describe purpose of culture.

2. Monitor technique of culture collection process for possible contamination.

3. Inspect specimen for traces of blood and reinspect mucosa if bleeding is apparent.

4. Ask client to describe comfort and anxiety levels.

Performance Checklist: Skill 14.6

Collecting a Sputum Specimen by Suction

	S	U	NP	Comments

Assessment

1. Check physician's orders for number and type of specimens needed. ____ ____ ____ _____

2. Assess client's understanding of procedure and its purpose. ____ ____ ____ _____

3. Assess client's ability to cough and expectorate sputum. ____ ____ ____ _____

4. Determine when client last ate a meal. ____ ____ ____ _____

5. Assess client's respiratory status. ____ ____ ____ _____

6. Assess client's anxiety level. ____ ____ ____ _____

Implementation

1. Use Standard Protocol. ____ ____ ____ _____

2. Position client in high or semi-Fowler's position. ____ ____ ____ _____

3. Explain procedure. ____ ____ ____ _____

4. Apply gloves. Prepare suction machine or device and determine whether it functions properly. ____ ____ ____ _____

5. Connect suction tube to adapter on sputum trap. ____ ____ ____ _____

6. Apply sterile gloves (required only for dominant hand). ____ ____ ____ _____

7. Preoxygenate for 1 minute with 100% oxygen. ____ ____ ____ _____

8. With gloved hand, connect sterile suction catheter to rubber tubing on sputum trap. ____ ____ ____ _____

9. Gently insert lubricated tip of suction catheter through nasopharynx, endotracheal tube, and tracheostomy without applying suction. ____ ____ ____ _____

10. Advance catheter into trachea. ____ ____ ____ _____

11. As client coughs, apply suction for 5 to 10 seconds, collecting 2 to 10 ml of sputum. ____ ____ ____ _____

		S	U	NP	Comments

	S	U	NP	Comments

12. Release suction and remove catheter, then turn off suction.

13. Detach catheter from specimen trap, and dispose of catheter into appropriate receptacle.

14. For sputum trap, detach suction tubing and connect rubber tubing on sputum trap to plastic adapter.

15. Wash off sputum on outside of container with disinfectant.

16. Offer client tissues and dispose after use.

17. Attach identification label and requisition to specimen container.

18. Enclose in plastic bag.

19. Send to laboratory immediately.

20. Offer client mouth care.

21. Use Completion Protocol.

Evaluation

1. Observe respiratory and oxygenation status throughout the procedure.

2. Ask client to describe the purpose and process of specimen collection.

3. Ask client to report level of comfort and anxiety.

4. Evaluate technique of collection process for sterility.

• Identify unexpected outcomes and intervene as necessary.

• Record and report intervention and client's response.

Performance Checklist: Procedural Guideline 14-4

Collecting a Sputum Specimen by Expectoration

		S	U	NP	Comments
1.	Use Standard Protocol.	___	___	___	_____
2.	Explain importance that client coughs and expectorates sputum.	___	___	___	_____
3.	Provide opportunity to cleanse or rinse mouth with water.	___	___	___	_____
4.	Apply gloves. Provide sputum cup and instruct client not to touch the inside of the container.	___	___	___	_____
5.	Have client take 3 or 4 deep breaths. Instruct client to emphasize slow, full exhalation. After a full exhalation, ask client to cough forcefully, expectorating sputum directly into specimen container.	___	___	___	_____
6.	Repeat until 5 to 10 ml of sputum, not saliva, has been collected.	___	___	___	_____
7.	Secure top on specimen container tightly. Wash off any sputum on the outside of container with a disinfectant.	___	___	___	_____
8.	Offer client tissues after expectorating, dispose of tissues, and offer mouth care.	___	___	___	_____
9.	Remove and dispose of gloves.	___	___	___	_____
10.	Securely attach properly completed label and requisition to specimen container.	___	___	___	_____
11.	Enclose specimen in a plastic bag.	___	___	___	_____
12.	Send specimen immediately to the laboratory.	___	___	___	_____
13.	Use Completion Protocol.	___	___	___	_____

Performance Checklist: Skill 14.7

Obtaining Wound Cultures

	S	U	NP	Comments

Assessment

1. Assess client for signs and symptoms of systemic infection.

2. Assess severity of pain at wound site.

3. Review physician's order for aerobic or anaerobic culture.

4. Determine when dressing change is scheduled.

5. Assess client's understanding of need for wound culture and ability to cooperate with procedure.

6. Apply clean gloves and remove any soiled dressing. Apply sterile gloves and inspect for swelling, opening of wound edges, inflammation, and drainage.

Implementation

1. Use Standard Protocol.

2. Apply gloves. Remove old dressing. Observe drainage. Fold soiled sides of dressing together and then dispose of in bag.

3. Cleanse area around wound edges with antiseptic swab. Remove old exudate.

4. Discard swab and dispose of soiled gloves in bag.

5. Open package containing sterile culture tube and dressing supplies.

6. Apply sterile gloves.

7. Obtain culture.
   a. Aerobic culture
      (1) Take swab from culture tube, insert tip into wound in area of drainage, and rotate swab gently.
      (2) Remove swab and return it to culture tube. Using a gauze pad between gloved fingers and the ampule, crush the ampule of medium and immediately push the swab into the fluid. Place top on culture tube securely.

	S	U	NP	Comments

b. Anaerobic culture: Take swab from special anaerobic culture tube, swab deeply into body cavity, and rotate gently. Remove swab and return to culture tube. Place top securely on tube.

OR

Insert tip of syringe (without needle) into wound and aspirate 5 to 10 ml of exudate. Attach 21-gauge needle, expel all air, and inject drainage into special culture tube. Clean wound as ordered, and apply new sterile dressing. Place top on culture tube securely.

8. Cleanse wound as ordered and apply new sterile dressing.

9. Ask another nurse or assistant to attach properly completed identification label and laboratory requisition to side of specimen container (not lid).

10. Enclose in plastic bag.

11. Send to laboratory immediately.

12. Remove and discard gloves.

13. Use Completion Protocol.

Evaluation

1. Ask client to rate pain level.

2. Observe character of wound drainage and note edges of wound.

3. Ask client to describe purpose of procedure.

4. Obtain laboratory report for results of cultures.

• Identify unexpected outcomes and intervene as necessary.

• Record and report intervention and client's response.

Performance Checklist: Skill 15.1

Intravenous Conscious Sedation

	S	U	NP	Comments

Assessment

1. Assess vital signs, electrocardiogram (ECG), level of consciousness, skin color, and presence of chest pain or shortness of breath.   ____ ____ ____ _____

2. Determine height and weight.   ____ ____ ____ _____

3. Assess respiratory status.   ____ ____ ____ _____

4. Palpate peripheral pulses and check for edema.   ____ ____ ____ _____

5. Determine time of last oral intake.   ____ ____ ____ _____

6. Assess level of anxiety.   ____ ____ ____ _____

Implementation

1. Use Standard Protocol.   ____ ____ ____ _____

2. Establish IV access.   ____ ____ ____ _____

3. Monitor and record vital signs every 5 to 15 minutes.   ____ ____ ____ _____

4. Observe for verbal or nonverbal evidence of pain.   ____ ____ ____ _____

5. Monitor level of consciousness and notify physician of acceptable scores.   ____ ____ ____ _____

6. Monitor ECG, oxygen saturation, and skin color.   ____ ____ ____ _____

7. Use Completion Protocol.   ____ ____ ____ _____

Evaluation

1. Ask client to explain purpose and basic steps of procedure.   ____ ____ ____ _____

2. Ask client to rate pain level.   ____ ____ ____ _____

3. Observe client for low oxygen saturation, respiratory function, cyanosis or mottled skin, hypotension, changes in heart rate or rhythm, and decreased peripheral pulses, reflexes, or level of consciousness.   ____ ____ ____ _____

• Identify unexpected outcomes and intervene as necessary.   ____ ____ ____ _____

• Record and report intervention and client's response.   ____ ____ ____ _____

Performance Checklist: Skill 15.2

Contrast Media Studies: Arteriogram, Cardiac Catheterization, Intravenous Pyelogram

	S	U	NP	Comments

Assessment

1. Assess client's knowledge of the procedure.

2. Observe verbal and nonverbal behaviors to determine level of client's anxiety.

3. Assess if client is allergic to iodine dye or shellfish; if so, notify cardiologist or radiologist.

4. Assess vital signs to provide baseline data for comparison with findings during and after procedure.

5. Assess peripheral pulses (for clients undergoing angiography) to provide baseline data for comparison with findings during and after procedure.

6. Assess hydration status of client.

7. Assess client's coagulation status.

8. Auscultate heart and lung sounds (for clients undergoing angiography) to provide baseline data for comparison with findings during and after procedure.

9. Verify that client has signed consent form (check institution policy).

10. Assess time of last ingested fluid or food.

11. Assess client's ability to remain still and cooperate throughout the procedure.

Implementation

1. Use Standard Protocol.

2. Assist client to empty bladder before procedure.

3. Assist with equipment application and setup for monitoring, if indicated.

4. Apply gloves. Establish IV access using large-bore cannula.

	S	U	NP	Comments

5. Assist client in assuming comfortable position on x-ray table.

6. Physician cleanses site for catheter insertion.

7. Apply sterile gown and gloves. Drape client with sterile drape.

8. Skin at puncture site is anesthetized.

9. Physician inserts needle and guide wire. Catheter is advanced and contrast medium injected.

10. Observe client for signs of anaphylaxis if iodinated dye administered.

11. Structures can be visualized as dye circulates.

12. Assist with measuring cardiac volumes and pressures during cardiac catheterization.

13. Physician withdraws catheter and applies pressure to site for 5 minutes.

14. Remove and discard gloves.

15. Keep client in position so insertion site extremity is kept straight. Client may remain in bed 4 to 6 hours.

16. Apply a pressure dressing or bandage over insertion site.

17. Use Completion Protocol.

Evaluation

1. Evaluate the client for understanding of and participation in the procedure.

2. Assess client's body position and comfort during procedure.

3. Ask if client has questions or concerns about the procedure or results.

4. Evaluate the client's comfort level.

5. Monitor vital signs every 15 minutes for 1 hour, then every 30 minutes for 2 hours or until vital signs are stable, then every 4 hours.

6. Monitor insertion site for bloody drainage or hematoma formation.

7. Assess neurovascular status in the affected extremity.

8. Auscultate heart and lungs and compare findings with baseline.

9. Monitor the client for allergic reactions.

	S	U	NP	Comments

10. Monitor client's level of consciousness and neurological status.

• Identify unexpected outcomes and intervene as necessary.

• Record and report intervention and client's response.

Performance Checklist: Skill 15.3

Assisting with Aspirations: Bone Marrow, Lumbar Puncture, Paracentesis, Thoracentesis

	S	U	NP	Comments

Assessment

1. Assess client's knowledge of procedure to determine level of health teaching required. ___ ___ ___ _____

2. Observe verbal and nonverbal behaviors to determine client's anxiety. ___ ___ ___ _____

3. Assess client's ability to understand and follow directions. ___ ___ ___ _____

4. Assess client's ability to assume position required for procedure and ability to remain still. ___ ___ ___ _____

5. Determine whether client is allergic to antiseptic or anesthetic solutions. ___ ___ ___ _____

6. Assess whether client has signed consent form (check institution's policy). ___ ___ ___ _____

7. Assess vital signs to provide baseline data for comparison with postprocedural vital signs. ___ ___ ___ _____

8. Assess client's coagulation status. ___ ___ ___ _____

9. Assess according to aspiration or diagnostic procedure being performed. ___ ___ ___ _____

10. Assess need for preprocedural pain medication. ___ ___ ___ _____

Implementation

1. Use Standard Protocol. ___ ___ ___ _____

2. Explain steps of skin preparation, anesthetic injection, needle insertion, and position required. ___ ___ ___ _____

3. Apply gloves. Set up sterile tray or open supplies to make accessible for physician. ___ ___ ___ _____

4. Obtain a premedication order if client is anxious. ___ ___ ___ _____

5. Assist client in maintaining correct position. Reassure client while explaining procedure. ___ ___ ___ _____

6. Physician cleanses and drapes site. ___ ___ ___ _____

	S	U	NP	Comments

7. Physician injects local anesthetic. ___ ___ ___ _____

8. Explain each step that may cause discomfort. ___ ___ ___ _____

9. Physician inserts trochar or needle. ___ ___ ___ _____

10. Syringe is attached to trochar or needle to aspire tissue or fluid. Aspirate placed into specimen container. ___ ___ ___ _____

11. Physician attaches drainage tubing and container if excess amount of fluid is to be drained. ___ ___ ___ _____

12. Properly label all specimens. ___ ___ ___ _____

13. Physician removes needle or trochar and applies pressure over site. Pressure dressing may be applied. ___ ___ ___ _____

14. Place antiseptic ointment with 2×2 gauze over site. ___ ___ ___ _____

15. Note characteristics of fluid or tissue. ___ ___ ___ _____

16. Remove and discard gloves. ___ ___ ___ _____

17. Use Completion Protocol. ___ ___ ___ _____

Evaluation

1. Evaluate the client for understanding of and participation in the procedure and position and activity restrictions. ___ ___ ___ _____

2. Ask if client has questions or concerns about the procedure or results. ___ ___ ___ _____

3. Observe body position throughout the procedure. ___ ___ ___ _____

4. Evaluate client's comfort level. ___ ___ ___ _____

5. Monitor respiratory status. Compare heart rate and blood pressure to baseline. ___ ___ ___ _____

6. Inspect dressing every hour after the procedure. ___ ___ ___ _____

7. Observe for postprocedural complications. ___ ___ ___ _____

8. Ask client to describe postprocedural positioning and activity restrictions. ___ ___ ___ _____

- Identify unexpected outcomes and intervene as necessary. ___ ___ ___ _____

- Record and report intervention and client's response. ___ ___ ___ _____

Name _____ Date _____ Instructor's Name _____

Performance Checklist: Skill 15.4

Assisting with Bronchoscopy

	S	U	NP	Comments

Assessment

1. Assess client's knowledge of procedure to determine level of health teaching required. ___ ___ ___ _____

2. Observe verbal and nonverbal behaviors to determine client's anxiety. ___ ___ ___ _____

3. Assess time of last ingested fluid or food. ___ ___ ___ _____

4. Assess vital signs to obtain baseline data. ___ ___ ___ _____

5. Assess client's allergies. ___ ___ ___ _____

6. Assess respiratory status. ___ ___ ___ _____

Implementation

1. Use Standard Protocol. ___ ___ ___ _____

2. Remove and safely store client's dentures and eyeglasses (if applicable). ___ ___ ___ _____

3. Apply gloves. Establish IV access using large-bore cannula. ___ ___ ___ _____

4. Assist client in maintaining desired position. ___ ___ ___ _____

5. Physician sprays nasopharynx and oropharynx with topical anesthetic. ___ ___ ___ _____

6. Instruct client not to swallow local anesthetic; provide emesis basin. ___ ___ ___ _____

7. Physician applies goggles, mask, and sterile gloves, and then introduces bronchoscope into mouth to pharynx to trachea and bronchi. ___ ___ ___ _____

8. Assist client through procedure by explanations. ___ ___ ___ _____

9. Monitor ECG, pulse, and blood pressure for changes every 5 minutes during procedure. ___ ___ ___ _____

10. Assess client's respiratory status every 5 minutes during procedure. ___ ___ ___ _____

11. Note characteristics of suctioned material. ___ ___ ___ _____

	S	U	NP	Comments

12. Wipe client's nose to remove lubricant after bronchoscope is removed.

13. Assess LOC, gag reflex, pulse oximetry, respiratory rate, blood pressure, pulse, heart rate, and capillary refill after the procedure.

14. Use tongue depressor to touch pharynx to test for return of gag reflex.

Nurse Alert: Do not allow client to eat or drink until the tracheobronchial anesthesia has worn off and gag reflex returns.

15. Remove and discard gloves.

16. Use Completion Protocol.

Evaluation

1. Monitor vital signs.

2. Observe character and amount of sputum.

3. Observe respiratory status closely.

4. Assess level of sedation and level of consciousness.

5. Monitor for return of gag reflex.

• Identify unexpected outcomes and intervene as necessary.

• Record and report intervention and client's response.

Performance Checklist: Skill 15.5

Assisting with Gastrointestinal Endoscopy: Esophagogastroduodenscopy

	S	U	NP	Comments

Assessment

1. Assess client's knowledge of procedure to determine level of health teaching required. ___ ___ ___ _____

2. Observe verbal and nonverbal behaviors to determine client's anxiety. ___ ___ ___ _____

3. Observe character of emesis, stool, and NB tube drainage for evidence of bleeding. ___ ___ ___ _____

4. Establish baseline vital signs. ___ ___ ___ _____

5. Verify that client has been NPO for at least 8 hours. ___ ___ ___ _____

6. Assess client's ability to understand and follow directions. ___ ___ ___ _____

Implementation

1. Use Standard Protocol. ___ ___ ___ _____

2. Remove client's dentures and partial bridges (if applicable). ___ ___ ___ _____

3. Monitor IV fluids and administer IVCS as ordered. ___ ___ ___ _____

4. Assist client through procedure by anticipating needs, promoting comfort, and telling client what is happening. ___ ___ ___ _____

5. Assist physician to spray nasopharynx and oropharynx with local anesthetic. ___ ___ ___ _____

6. Position client in left lateral position. ___ ___ ___ _____

7. Physician passes endoscope into mouth, esophagus, stomach, or duodenum, examines structures, and performs biopsy, if appropriate. ___ ___ ___ _____

8. Place tissue specimens in properly labeled laboratory containers. ___ ___ ___ _____

9. Suction if client begins to vomit or accumulate saliva. ___ ___ ___ _____

10. Inform client not to eat or drink until gag reflex returns. ___ ___ ___ _____

	S	U	NP	Comments

11. Use Completion Protocol. ___ ___ ___ _____

Evaluation

1. Evaluate client's understanding of the procedure. ___ ___ ___ _____

2. Observe for verbal and nonverbal signs of fear and anxiety. ___ ___ ___ _____

3. Observe positioning and ability to cooperate throughout the procedure. ___ ___ ___ _____

4. Ask client to evaluate comfort level. ___ ___ ___ _____

5. Observe for return of gag reflex if local anesthetic is used. ___ ___ ___ _____

6. Monitor vital signs. ___ ___ ___ _____

- Identify unexpected outcomes and intervene as necessary. ___ ___ ___ _____

- Record and report intervention and client's response. ___ ___ ___ _____

Performance Checklist: Procedural Guideline 15-1

Assisting with Colonoscopy

	S	U	NP	Comments
1. Use Standard Protocol.	___	___	___	_____
2. Instruct client in preparation. Lower GI tract is cleansed by maintaining a liquid diet for 2 days before the procedure. One day prior to the test, the client takes a chilled electrolyte laxative solution, usually 8 ounces every 15 minutes until 1 gallon is ingested.	___	___	___	_____
3. Premedicate client with narcotic as ordered. IV conscious sedation may be used.	___	___	___	_____
4. Assist in positioning the client on the left side, with legs and hips flexed.	___	___	___	_____
5. Apply gloves. Physician inserts scope through rectum and sigmoid, descending, transverse, and ascending colons.	___	___	___	_____
6. Air is instilled to distend the colon as the scope is advanced.	___	___	___	_____
7. Biopsy forceps and cytology brush may be used to obtain specimens. Complete laboratory slips and send specimens to the laboratory.	___	___	___	_____
8. Scope is removed and rectal area cleaned and dried.	___	___	___	_____
9. See Completion Protocol.	___	___	___	_____

Performance Checklist: Skill 15.6

Assisting with Electrocardiograms

	S	U	NP	Comments

Assessment

1. Assess client's knowledge of the procedure to determine level of health teaching required. _____ _____ _____ _____

2. Observe verbal and nonverbal behaviors to determine client's anxiety. _____ _____ _____ _____

3. Assess client's ability to understand and follow directions. _____ _____ _____ _____

Implementation

1. Use Standard Protocol. _____ _____ _____ _____

2. Expose client's chest and arms and cleanse and prepare skin; wipe sites with alcohol. _____ _____ _____ _____

3. If large amounts of hair are present, it may be necessary to clip the hair at the placement sites. _____ _____ _____ _____

4. Apply self-sticking electrodes or electrode paste and attach leads. For 12-lead ECG:
   a. Chest (precordial leads)
      (1) V1—4th intercostal space (ICS) at right sternal border _____ _____ _____ _____
      (2) V2—4th ICS at left sternal border _____ _____ _____ _____
      (3) V3—midway between V2 and V4 _____ _____ _____ _____
      (4) V4—5th ICS at midclavicular line _____ _____ _____ _____
      (5) V5—left anterior axillary line at level of V4 horizontally _____ _____ _____ _____
      (6) V6—left midaxillary line at level of V4 horizontally _____ _____ _____ _____
   b. Extremities: one on lower portion of each extremity
      (1) aV_R—right wrist _____ _____ _____ _____
      (2) aV_L—left wrist _____ _____ _____ _____
      (3) aV_F—left ankle _____ _____ _____ _____

5. Turn on machine and obtain tracing; 12-lead ECG may be obtained without removing precordial leads. Ask client to lie quietly until a reading is obtained. _____ _____ _____ _____

6. Disconnect leads, wipe excess electrode paste from chest, and wash hands. _____ _____ _____ _____

	S	U	NP	Comments

7. Deliver ECG tracing to appropriate
   laboratory or nursing unit.   ___ ___ ___ _____

8. Use Completion Protocol.   ___ ___ ___ _____

Evaluation

1. Ask client to explain the procedure.   ___ ___ ___ _____

2. Discuss anxiety and fears related to test
   process and results.   ___ ___ ___ _____

3. Observe client's ability to understand and
   follow directions.   ___ ___ ___ _____

4. Determine client's ability to maintain
   position required for procedure.   ___ ___ ___ _____

- Identify unexpected outcomes and intervene
  as necessary.   ___ ___ ___ _____

- Record and report intervention and client's
  response.   ___ ___ ___ _____

Performance Checklist: Skill 17.1

Administering Oral Medications

	S	U	NP	Comments

Assessment

1. Identify the drug(s) ordered: action, purpose, normal dosage and route, common side effects, time of onset and peak action, and nursing implications.

2. Assess for any contraindications to oral medication.

3. Check allergies and replace any missing or faded identification bracelets.

4. Check for ID band or photograph.

5. Assess client's knowledge regarding medications.

6. Assess client's preferences for fluids. Maintain fluid restrictions as prescribed.

Implementation

1. Use Standard Protocol.

2. Prepare medications
   a. Compare medication administration record with scheduled medication list. If discrepancies exist, check against original physician orders.

Nurse Alert: Clarify incomplete or unclear orders with the prescriber.

   b. Arrange cups in medication preparation area or move medication cart to position outside client's room.
   c. Unlock medicine drawer or cart.
   d. Prepare medications for one client at a time.
   e. Select correct drug from stock supply or unit dose drawer. Compare label of medication with MAR or computer printout.
   f. Check drug dose. If label dose differs from ordered dose, calculate correct amount to give.

g. To prepare unit dose tablets or capsules, place packaged tablet or capsule directly into medicine cup without removing wrapper. ____ ____ ____ _____

h. To prepare tablets or capsules from a floor stock bottle, pour required number into bottle cap and transfer medication to medication cup. Do not touch medication with fingers; return extra tablets or capsules to bottle. ____ ____ ____ _____

i. Check the expiration date of each drug. Return all outdated drugs to pharmacy. ____ ____ ____ _____

j. Place all tablets or capsules requiring preadministration assessments (e.g., pulse rate, blood pressure) in a separate cup. ____ ____ ____ _____

k. Medications that need to, and can be, broken in order to administer half the dose can be broken using a gloved hand or cut with a cutting device. ____ ____ ____ _____

l. When using a blister pack, pop medications through a foil or paper backing into a medication cup. ____ ____ ____ _____

m. When preparing liquids, thoroughly mix before administering, and discard medications that are cloudy or have changed color.
   (1) Place cap upside down while pouring. ____ ____ ____ _____
   (2) Hold label against palm of hand while pouring. ____ ____ ____ _____
   (3) Place medication cup at eye level and fill to desired level. ____ ____ ____ _____
   (4) Wipe lip of bottle with paper towel. ____ ____ ____ _____
   (5) If giving less than 5 ml of liquids, prepare medication in a sterile syringe without a needle. Give cold carbonated water if available and not contraindicated. ____ ____ ____ _____

n. If client has difficulty swallowing, use a mortar and pestle to grind pills or a pill-crushing device. Mix ground tablet in small amount of soft food. ____ ____ ____ _____

Nurse Alert: Not all drugs can be crushed. Consult with pharmacist when in doubt or to determine whether there is a liquid or suppository form available.

o. Narcotic preparation. Check narcotic record for previous drug count and compare with supply available. ____ ____ ____ _____

p. Check expiration date on all medications. ____ ____ ____ _____

3. Administer medications
   a. Take medications to client within 30 minutes before or after scheduled time. ____ ____ ____ _____

	S	U	NP	Comments

b. Identify client.

c. Perform necessary preadministration assessment for specific medications.

d. Discuss the purpose of each medication and its action with client. Allow client to ask any questions about drugs.

e. Assist client to sitting or side-lying position.

Nurse Alert: Check ability to swallow if appropriate.

f. Client may wish to hold solid medications in hand or cup before placing in mouth.

g. If client is unable to hold medications, place medication cup to the lips and gently introduce each drug into the mouth, one at a time. Do not rush.

h. Offer water or juice to help client to swallow medications.

i. For sublingually administered drugs, have client place medication under tongue and allow it to dissolve completely. Caution client against swallowing tablet.

j. For buccally administered drugs, have client place medication in mouth against mucous membranes of the cheek until it dissolves.

Nurse Alert: Decide on sequence of administration if client is receiving a combination of oral medication types.

k. Mix powdered medications with liquids at bedside and give to client to drink.

l. Caution client against chewing or swallowing lozenges.

m. Give effervescent powders and tablets immediately after dissolving.

n. Stay until client has completely swallowed each medication. If concerned about ability or willingness to swallow, ask client to open mouth and inspect for presence of medication.

o. For certain medications that should not be given on an empty stomach, offer client nonfat snack.

4. Replenish stock such as cups and straws, return cart to medicine room, and clean work area.

5. Use Completion Protocol.

	S	U	NP	Comments

Evaluation

1. Return within appropriate time to determine client's response to medications.

2. Evaluate client's or family member's learning needs.

- Identify unexpected outcomes and intervene as necessary.

- Record and report intervention and client's response.

Performance Checklist: Skill 17.2

Applying Topical Medications

	S	U	NP	Comments

Assessment

1. Review physician's order for client's name, name of drug, strength, time of administration, and site of application.

2. Review information pertinent to medication: action, purpose, side effects, and nursing implications.

3. Assess condition of client's skin. Cleanse skin if necessary to visualize adequately.

4. Determine whether client has known allergy to latex or topical agent.

5. Determine amount of topical agent required for application.

6. Determine whether client is physically able to apply medication.

Implementation

1. Use Standard Protocol.

Nurse Alert: Apply the six "rights" of drug administration.

2. Apply topical creams, ointments, and oil-based lotions.
   a. Wear gloves. Expose affected area while keeping unaffected areas covered.
   b. Wash affected area, removing all debris, encrustations, and previous medication.
   c. Soak area with plain warm water to removed crusted tissues.
   d. Pat skin or allow to air dry.
   e. If skin is excessively dry and flaking, apply topical agent while skin is still damp.
   f. Remove gloves, and apply new clean gloves.
   g. Place approximately 1 to 2 teaspoons of medication in palm of gloved hand and soften by rubbing briskly between hands.
   h. Once medication is thin and smooth, smear it evenly over skin surface, using

long, even strokes that follow direction
of hair growth.   ___ ___ ___ _____

  i. Explain to client that skin may feel greasy.   ___ ___ ___ _____

3. Apply antianginal (nitroglycerin) ointment.
  a. Apply gloves. Remove previous dosage
paper.   ___ ___ ___ _____

  b. Apply desired number of inches of
ointment over paper measuring guide.   ___ ___ ___ _____

  c. Antianginal (nitroglycerin) ointments are
usually ordered in inches and can be
measured on small sheets of paper
marked off in 1/2-inch markings. Unit
dose packages are available.   ___ ___ ___ _____

  d. Antianginal medication may be applied
to the chest area, back, upper arm, or legs.
Do not apply on hairy surfaces or over
scar tissue.   ___ ___ ___ _____

  e. Be sure to rotate sites.   ___ ___ ___ _____

  f. Apply ointment to skin surface by holding
edge or back of the paper wrapper and
placing ointment and wrapper directly
on the skin.   ___ ___ ___ _____

  g. Do not rub or massage ointment into skin.   ___ ___ ___ _____

  h. Date, time, and initial paper and note time.   ___ ___ ___ _____

  i. Cover ointment and paper with plastic
wrap and tape securely, or follow
manufacturer's directions. Discard gloves
and wash hands.   ___ ___ ___ _____

4. Apply transdermal patches (e.g., analgesic,
nitroglycerin, nicotine, estrogen).
  a. Choose a clean, dry area of the body that
is free of hair.   ___ ___ ___ _____

**Nurse Alert: It is recommended that nitroglycerin
patches be removed after 10 to 12 hours. Check
with prescriber. Estrogen patches should never be
applied to breast tissue.**

  b. Apply gloves. Carefully remove the patch
from its protective covering. Hold the
patch by the edge.   ___ ___ ___ _____

  c. Immediately apply the patch, pressing
firmly with the palm of one hand for 10
seconds. Make sure it sticks well, especially
around the edges. Date and initial patch
and note time.   ___ ___ ___ _____

  d. Advise clients not to use heating pads
anywhere near the site.   ___ ___ ___ _____

  e. After appropriate time, remove the patch
and fold it so the medicated side is
covered, and discard appropriately.
Discard gloves and wash hands.   ___ ___ ___ _____

    f. Avoid previously used sites for at least 1 week.

5. Administer aerosol spray.
    a. Shake container vigorously.
    b. Read container's label for distance recommended to hold spray away from area, usually 6 to 12 inches (15-30 cm).
    c. If neck or upper chest is to be sprayed, ask client to turn face away from spray or briefly cover face with towel.
    d. Spray medication evenly over affected site (in some cases, spray is timed for period of seconds).

6. Apply suspension-based lotion.
    a. Shake container vigorously.
    b. Apply small amount of lotion to small gauze dressing or pad, and apply to skin by stroking evenly in direction of hair growth.
    c. Explain to client that area will feel cool and dry.

7. Apply medicated powder.
    a. Be sure skin surface is thoroughly dry.
    b. Fully spread apart any skinfolds such as between toes or under axillae.
    c. Dust skin site lightly with dispenser so that area is covered with fine, thin layer of powder.
    d. Cover skin area with dressing if ordered by physician.

8. Instruct client to dispose of applicators, patches, and similar materials into cardboard or plastic disposable containers.

9. Use Completion Protocol.

Evaluation

1. Evaluate condition of skin.

2. Observe client's ability to apply medication.

3. Evaluate learning needs of client and family.

• Identify unexpected outcomes and intervene as necessary.

• Record and report intervention and client's response.

Performance Checklist: Skill 17.3

Instilling Eye and Ear Medications

	S	U	NP	Comments

Assessment

1. Review physician's medication order, including client's name, drug name, concentration, number of drops (if a liquid), time, and eye or ear.

2. Review information pertinent to medication, including action, purpose, side effects, and nursing implications.

3. Assess condition of external eye or ear structures.

4. Determine whether client has symptoms of discomfort or hearing or visual impairment.

5. Determine whether client has any known allergies to medications.

6. Assess client's level of consciousness and ability to follow directions.

7. Assess client's knowledge regarding drug therapy and desire to self-administer medication.

8. Assess client's ability to manipulate and hold dropper.

Implementation

1. Use Standard Protocol.

2. Compare MAR with label of medication. Review the six "rights" of medication administration.

3. Verify client's identification.

4. Explain procedure to client. Clients experienced in self-instillation may be allowed to give drops under nurse's supervision (check agency policy).

5. Apply gloves. Ask client to lie supine or sit back in chair with neck slightly hyperextended for eye drops. For ear drops, position client on side or sitting in chair with affected ear

	S	U	NP	Comments

facing up. Gently wash away drainage from inner to outer canthus.

Nurse Alert: Do not hyperextend the neck of a client with a cervical spine injury.

6. Instill eye drops
   a. Apply glove. Hold cotton ball or clean tissue in nondominant hand on client's cheekbone just below lower eyelid.
   b. With tissue or cotton resting below lower lid, gently press downward with thumb or forefinger against bony orbit, exposing conjunctival sac.
   c. Ask client to look at ceiling.
   d. Rest dominant hand gently on client's forehead, and hold filled medication eyedropper approximately ½ to ¾ inch (1-2 cm) into conjunctival sac.
   e. Drop prescribed number of medication drops into conjunctival sac.
   f. If client blinks or closes eye or if drops land on outer lid margins, repeat procedure.
   g. When administering drugs that cause systemic effects, apply gentle pressure to client's nasolacrimal duct with cotton ball or tissue for 30 to 60 seconds.
   h. After instilling drops, ask client to close eye gently.

7. To instill eye ointment:
   a. Apply gloves. Ask client to look up.
   b. Apply thin stream of ointment along upper lid margin on inner conjunctiva.
   c. Have client close eye and rub lid lightly in circular motion with cotton ball, if rubbing is not contraindicated.
   d. If excess medication is on eyelid, gently wipe it from inner to outer canthus.

8. If client needs an eye patch, apply clean one by placing it over affected eye so entire eye is covered. Tape securely without applying pressure to eye.

9. Intraocular disk application
   a. Open package containing the disk. Gently press your fingertip against the disk so that it adheres to your finger. Position the convex side of the disk on you fingertip.
   b. With your other hand, gently pull the client's lower eyelid away from the eye. Ask client to look up.

	S	U	NP	Comments

c. Place the disk in the conjunctival sac, so that it floats on the sclera between the iris and lower eyelid. ___ ___ ___ _____

d. Pull the client's lower eyelid out and over the disk. Repeat if disk is seen. ___ ___ ___ _____

10. Removal of intraocular disk
  a. Gently pull on the client's lower eyelid to expose the disk. ___ ___ ___ _____
  b. Using your forefinger and thumb of your opposite hand, pinch the disk and lift it out of the client's eye. ___ ___ ___ _____
  c. If excess medication is on eyelid, gently wipe it from inner to outer canthus. ___ ___ ___ _____
  d. If client had eye patch, apply clean one by placing it over affected eye so entire eye is covered. Tape securely without applying pressure to eye. ___ ___ ___ _____

11. Instill ear drops
  a. Apply gloves if drainage is present.
  b. Warm ear drops to body temperature. Hold bottle in hands or place in warm water. Position client with affected ear facing up. ___ ___ ___ _____
  c. Straighten ear canal by pulling auricle upward and outward (adult) or down and back (child). ___ ___ ___ _____
  d. If cerumen or drainage occludes outermost portion of ear canal, wipe out gently with cotton-tipped applicator, taking care not to force wax inward. ___ ___ ___ _____
  e. Instill prescribed drops holding dropper 1/2 inch (1 cm) above ear canal. ___ ___ ___ _____
  f. Ask client to remain in side-lying position 5 to 10 minutes, and apply gentle massage or pressure to tragus of ear with finger. ___ ___ ___ _____
  g. If ordered, gently insert a portion of cotton ball into outermost part of canal. ___ ___ ___ _____
  h. Remove cotton after 15 minutes. ___ ___ ___ _____

12. Use Completion Protocol. ___ ___ ___ _____

Evaluation

1. Evaluate effects of the medication. ___ ___ ___ _____

2. Note client's response to instillation and observe for side effects. ___ ___ ___ _____

3. Ask client to discuss medication—purpose, side effects, and technique of administration. ___ ___ ___ _____

		S	U	NP	Comments
4.	Evaluate client's ability to self-administer.	___	___	___	_____
•	Identify unexpected outcomes and intervene as necessary.	___	___	___	_____
•	Record and report intervention and client's response.	___	___	___	_____

Name _____ Date _____ Instructor's Name _____

Performance Checklist: Skill 17.4

Using Metered-Dose Inhalers

	S	U	NP	Comments

Assessment

1. Assess respiratory pattern and auscultate breath sounds.

2. Assess client's ability to hold, manipulate, and depress canister and inhaler.

3. Assess client's readiness to learn.

4. Assess client's ability to learn.

5. Assess client's knowledge and understanding of disease and purpose and action of prescribed medications.

6. Identify medication order, drug schedule, and number of inhalations prescribed for each dose.

Implementation

1. Use Standard Protocol.

Nurse Alert: Review the six "rights" of medication administration.

2. Allow client opportunity to manipulate inhaler, canister, and spacer device (aerochamber). Explain and demonstrate how canister fits into inhaler.

3. Explain what metered dose is, and warn client about overuse of inhaler, including drug side effects.

4. Remove mouth piece cover from inhaler.

5. Shake inhaler well.

6. Without aerochamber (spacer): Have client take a deep breath and exhale completely. Instruct client to open lips and place inhaler $\frac{1}{2}$ to 1 inch (1-2 cm) from mouth with opening toward back of throat. Lips should not touch inhaler.

7. With spacer device: Have client exhale fully, then grasp spacer mouthpiece with teeth and lips while holding inhaler with thumb

at the mouthpiece and fingers at the
top of the inhaler.

8. Instruct client to tilt head back slightly and
press down on inhaler to release medication
while inhaling slowly and deeply through
mouth.

9. Ask client to breathe in slowly for 2 to 3
seconds. Hold breath for approximately 10
seconds.

10. Have client exhale through pursed lips.

11. Instruct client to wait 2 to 5 minutes
between puffs. More than one puff is
usually prescribed.

12. If more than one type of inhaled medication
is prescribed, wait 5 to 10 minutes between
inhalations or as ordered by physician.

13. Instruct client to rinse mouth after
steroid administration. Instruct client to
remove medication canister and clean
inhaler in warm water after each use.

14. Instruct client against repeating inhalations
before next scheduled dose.

15. Teach client to measure the amount of
medication remaining in the canister by
immersing it in a large bowl or pan of water.

16. Use Completion Protocol.

Evaluation

1. Have client explain and demonstrate the use
of the inhaler.

2. Ask client to explain drug schedule and dose.

3. Assess respirations and auscultate lungs.

4. Assess knowledge of side effects and when to
call the physician.

• Identify unexpected outcomes and intervene
as necessary.

• Record and report intervention and client's
response.

Performance Checklist: Skill 17.5

Using Small-Volume Nebulizers

	S	U	NP	Comments

Assessment

1. Assess client's medical history, allergies, and medications.

2. Assess client's ability to hold and manipulate the nebulizer equipment.

3. Assess drug ordered.

4. Assess pulse, respirations, and breath sounds before beginning treatment.

Implementation

1. Use Standard Protocol.

Nurse Alert: Review the six "rights" of medication administration.

2. Explain the use of the nebulizer and possible drug side effects.

Nurse Alert: Administer respiratory drugs with systemic effects with caution to clients with cardiac disease. Discontinue the drug and notify the physician immediately if bronchospasm occurs during treatment.

3. Assemble the nebulizer equipment per manufacturer's instructions.

4. Add the prescribed medication and diluent to the nebulizer.

5. Have client hold the mouthpiece between the lips with gentle pressure.
   a. A face mask may be used for a child, infant, or adult who is fatigued or cannot follow instructions.
   b. Special adapters are used for clients with tracheostomies.

6. Have client take a deep breath slowly to a volume slightly greater than normal. After inspiration, have the client pause briefly, then have the client exhale passively.
   a. If client is dyspneic, encourage client to hold every fourth or fifth breath for 5 to 10 seconds.

7. Turn on the small volume nebulizer machine and ensure that a sufficient mist is formed.
   a. Tap the nebulizer cup occasionally during and near the end of treatment.   ____ ____ ____ _____
   b. Remind client to repeat the breathing pattern in step 7 until the drug is completely nebulized. A length of treatment time may be specified by the prescriber.
   c. Monitor client's pulse.   ____ ____ ____ _____

8. When medication is completely nebulized or the time has ended, turn off the machine and store the tubing assembly per agency policy.
   a. Shake the nebulizer bottle to remove remaining solution. Never rinse with tap water.   ____ ____ ____ _____
   b. Teach client not to store medication in nebulizer for later use.   ____ ____ ____ _____

9. Encourage client to rinse mouth and gargle with warm water if steroids are nebulized.   ____ ____ ____ _____

10. Use Completion Protocol.   ____ ____ ____ _____

Evaluation

1. Assess client's pulse, respiratory rate, and breath sounds after procedure.   ____ ____ ____ _____

2. Ask client to explain use of small-volume nebulizer.   ____ ____ ____ _____

3. Observe while client self-administers medication with nebulizer.   ____ ____ ____ _____

4. Ask client to explain and demonstrate care of nebulizer.   ____ ____ ____ _____

5. Ask client to describe side effects of medications and when to call the physician.   ____ ____ ____ _____

• Identify unexpected outcomes and intervene as necessary.   ____ ____ ____ _____

• Record and report intervention and client's response.   ____ ____ ____ _____

Name _____ Date _____ Instructor's Name _____

Performance Checklist: Skill 17.6

Inserting Rectal and Vaginal Medications

	S	U	NP	Comments

Assessment

1. Review physician's order, including client's name, drug name, form (cream or suppository), route, dosage, and time of administration. ____ ____ ____ _____

2. Review pertinent information related to medication, including action, purpose, side effects, and nursing implications. ____ ____ ____ _____

3. Inspect condition of external genitalia and vaginal canal or rectum. (May be done just before insertion.) ____ ____ ____ _____

4. Ask if client is experiencing any symptoms of pruritus, burning, bleeding, or discomfort. ____ ____ ____ _____

5. Review client's knowledge of purpose of drug therapy and ability and willingness to self-administer medication. ____ ____ ____ _____

6. Review medical record for history of rectal surgery or bleeding. ____ ____ ____ _____

Implementation

1. Use Standard Protocol. ____ ____ ____ _____

Nurse Alert: Review the six "rights" of medication administration.

2. Administer rectal suppository
   a. Apply gloves. Assist client in assuming a left side-lying Sims' position with upper leg flexed upward. ____ ____ ____ _____
   b. Keep client covered with only anal area exposed. ____ ____ ____ _____
   c. Examine condition of anus externally and palpate rectal walls as needed. ____ ____ ____ _____

Nurse Alert: Do not palpate client's rectum after rectal surgery. Use a liberal amount of lubricant for clients with hemorrhoids. Rectal suppositories are contraindicated in the presence of active bleeding or diarrhea.

   d. Apply clean disposable gloves (if previous gloves were soiled and discarded). ____ ____ ____ _____

e. Remove suppository from foil wrapper
and lubricate rounded end.
_____ _____ _____ _____

f. Retract client's buttocks with
nondominant hand. Ask client to take
slow, deep breaths through mouth and to
relax anal sphincter.
_____ _____ _____ _____

g. With gloved index finger of dominant
hand, insert suppository, rounded end
first, gently through anus, past internal
sphincter, and against rectal wall, 4 inches
(10 cm) in adults.
_____ _____ _____ _____

h. Wipe client's anal area and discard gloves
by turning them inside out, and dispose
of in appropriate receptacle.
_____ _____ _____ _____

i. Ask client to remain on side for 5 to 10
minutes or until urge to eliminate is
strong.
_____ _____ _____ _____

j. If suppository contains laxative or fecal
softener, place call light within reach so
client can obtain assistance to reach
bedpan or toilet.
_____ _____ _____ _____

3. Administer vaginal suppository.
   a. Apply gloves. Assist client to lie in dorsal
   recumbent position with abdomen and
   lower extremities covered.
   _____ _____ _____ _____

   b. Be sure vaginal orifice is well illuminated.
   _____ _____ _____ _____

   c. Remove suppository from foil wrapper
   and apply liberal amount of petroleum
   jelly. Lubricate gloved finger.
   _____ _____ _____ _____

   d. With nondominant gloved hand, gently
   retract labial folds to expose vaginal
   orifice.
   _____ _____ _____ _____

   e. Insert rounded end of suppository along
   posterior wall of vaginal canal 3 to 4 inches
   (7.5-10 cm).
   _____ _____ _____ _____

   f. Wipe away remaining lubricant from
   around orifice and labia. Remove and
   discard gloves.
   _____ _____ _____ _____

   g. Tell client there may be a small amount
   of discharge that is the color of medication
   exiting from vaginal canal. Client may
   wish to use disposable panty liners.
   _____ _____ _____ _____

4. Administer vaginal cream or foam.
   a. Apply gloves. Fill cream or foam
   applicator following package directions.
   _____ _____ _____ _____

   b. With nondominant gloved hand, gently
   retract labial folds to expose vaginal
   orifice.
   _____ _____ _____ _____

   c. With dominant gloved hand, insert
   applicator approximately 2 to 3 inches
   (5-7.5 cm). Push applicator plunger to
   deposit medication into vagina.
   _____ _____ _____ _____

	S	U	NP	Comments

d. Withdraw applicator and place on paper towel. Wipe off residual cream from labia or vaginal orifice.

e. Instruct client who received suppository or cream to remain supine for at least 10 minutes.

f. Offer disposable panty liners for use during ambulation.

5. Use Completion Protocol.

Evaluation

1. Ask client about relief of symptoms.

2. Monitor condition of external genitalia or rectum.

3. Evaluate client's understanding of and response to medication.

• Identify unexpected outcomes and intervene as necessary.

• Record and report intervention and client's response.

Performance Checklist: Procedure Guideline 18-1

Reconstituting Medications from a Powder

	S	U	NP	Comments
1. Remove cap covering vial containing powdered medication and vial containing diluent. Label may specify use of sterile water, normal saline, or special diluent provided with the medication.	___	___	___	_____
2. Firmly swab both caps with alcohol swab and allow to dry.	___	___	___	_____
3. Draw up diluent into syringe with needle.	___	___	___	_____
4. Insert tip of needle through center of rubber seal of vial of powdered medication and inject diluent into vial.	___	___	___	_____
5. Remove needle.	___	___	___	_____
6. Mix medication by gently rolling vial between hands until completely dissolved.	___	___	___	_____
7. Reconstituted medication in vial is ready to be drawn into syringe. Read label carefully to determine concentration after reconstitution.	___	___	___	_____
8. Draw up medication into syringe.	___	___	___	_____

Performance Checklist: Procedure Guideline 18-2

Mixing Medications from a Vial

	S	U	NP	Comments
1. Remove protective covering from top of vials and cleanse tops of both vials with alcohol swab.	___	___	___	_____
2. Take syringe with needle and aspirate volume of air equivalent to first medication's dosage (vial A).	___	___	___	_____
3. Inject air into vial A, making sure needle does not touch solution. Withdraw needle.	___	___	___	_____
4. Repeat with vial B. Without removing needle from vial B, fill syringe with proper volume of medication.	___	___	___	_____
5. Calculate total volume of medication by adding volume of both prescribed medications.	___	___	___	_____
6. Insert needle of syringe into vial A, being careful not to push plunger and expel medication into vial. Invert vial and carefully withdraw the exact amount of medication required into the syringe.	___	___	___	_____

Performance Checklist: Skill 18.1

Subcutaneous Injections (Includes Insulin)

	S	U	NP	Comments

Assessment

1. Review physician's orders for client's name, drug name, dose, and time and route of administration.

2. Gather information pertinent to drug(s) ordered.

3. Check expiration date of medication.

4. Assess for factors that may contraindicate subcutaneous (SQ) injections.

5. Assess indications for SQ injections.

6. Assess client's medical history, history of allergies, and medication history.

7. Assess adequacy of adipose tissue.

8. Assess client's knowledge regarding medication to be received.

9. Observe client's verbal and nonverbal response toward injection.

10. Ask if client prefers to administer own injection if accustomed to doing so. If learning to do own injections, reinforce learning process.

Implementation

1. Use Standard Protocol.

Nurse Alert: Review the six "rights" of medication administration.

2. Prepare medication in syringe.

3. Identity client.

4. Provide privacy. Explain procedure.

5. Select appropriate injection site. Inspect skin's surface over sites for bruises, inflammation, edema, or tenderness.

6. Be sure needle size is correct by grasping skinfold at site with thumb and forefinger. Measure skinfold from top to bottom, and

be sure needle is approximately half this
length.

7. Assist client to comfortable position and ask
client to relax arm, leg, or abdomen,
depending on site chosen for injection.

8. Talk with client about subject of interest.
Keep needle out of line of vision.

9. Apply gloves. Relocate site using anatomical
landmarks.

10. Cleanse site with an antiseptic swab. Apply
swab to the center of the site and rotate
outward in a circular direction for about 2
inches (5 cm).

11. Hold swab or square of gauze between
fingers of nondominant hand or place near
site.

12. Remove needle cap or sheath from needle
by pulling it straight off.

13. Hold syringe between thumb and forefinger
of dominant hand as if grasping dart or
hold syringe across tops of fingertips.

14. Administer injection.
    a. Average size client: Spread skin tightly or
       pinch skin and inject needle quickly and
       firmly at a 90-degree angle.
    b. Thin client or child: Gently pinch skin
       and inject needle quickly and firmly at
       45-degree angle using a $\frac{1}{2}$- to $\frac{5}{16}$-inch
       needle.
    c. Obese client: Pinch skin at site and inject
       needle at a 90-degree angle below tissue
       fold.

15. After needle enters site, grasp lower end of
syringe barrel with nondominant hand.
Move dominant hand to end of plunger.
Avoid moving syringe.

Nurse Alert: Do not aspirate medication.

16. With dominant hand, inject medication
slowly but smoothly.

**Nurse Alert: Injecting heparin over 30 seconds
may create less painful bruising.**

17. Withdraw needle quickly while placing
antiseptic swab or gauze gently above or
over site.

18. Apply gentle pressure to site. Do not
massage site.

	S	U	NP	Comments

19. Discard uncapped needle or needle enclosed in safety shield in appropriately labeled receptacle.   _____ _____ _____   _____

20. Use Completion Protocol.   _____ _____ _____   _____

Evaluation

1. Evaluate client's response to medication after injection to determine effectiveness of drug and undesired side effects.   _____ _____ _____   _____

2. Ask if client feels burning, numbness, or tingling at the injection site.   _____ _____ _____   _____

3. Inspect and palpate site for lumps, tenderness, or swelling.   _____ _____ _____   _____

4. Ask client to describe medication.   _____ _____ _____   _____

For insulin
5. Monitor blood glucose level.   _____ _____ _____   _____

6. Ask client to list symptoms of hypoglycemia and hyperglycemia.   _____ _____ _____   _____

For heprain
7. Have client describe signs of bleeding to report.   _____ _____ _____   _____

8. Routinely monitor for thrombus formation and bleeding.   _____ _____ _____   _____

- Identify unexpected outcomes and intervene as necessary.   _____ _____ _____   _____

- Record and report intervention and client's response.   _____ _____ _____   _____

Name _____ Date _____ Instructor's Name _____

Performance Checklist: Procedural Guideline 18-3

Teaching Self-Injections

		S	U	NP	Comments
1.	Determine whether client is ready and able to learn this skill.				
2.	Determine client's ability to read and see medication label and syringe markings clearly.				
3.	Assess client's ability to hold and manipulate a syringe and vial.				
4.	Include significant other in teaching if possible.				
5.	Assemble teaching materials and equipment needed. Provide a comfortable, quiet, well-lit setting, free of distractions. Have client sit at table where equipment is displayed, making sure equipment is within easy reach.				
6.	Describe appropriate storage of medication and supplies.				
7.	Have client wash hands. Explain importance of hand washing.				
8.	Have client manipulate syringe. Explain sterile technique.				
9.	Discuss medication dosage and show client how much to draw up into syringe.				
10.	Have client wipe off top of medication vial or vials with alcohol swab. Explain purpose of this action.				
11.	Have client remove needle cover and pull plunger out to same amount of medication to be removed from vial.				
12.	With vial still on table, have client push needle slowly into rubber on top of vial while holding syringe barrel carefully.				
13.	Instruct client to push in plunger to push air into vial.				
14.	Holding vial and syringe together, instruct client to turn both upside down. Hold vial between thumb and forefinger, supporting syringe with other hand.				

15. Teach client to slowly pull back on plunger until the correct amount of medication is transferred into the syringe. Be sure client keeps the needle under the fluid level in the vial. ____ ____ ____ _____

16. Have client check for and remove air bubbles inside syringe. To clear bubbles, the client should tap lightly and expel them back into the vial. Before withdrawing the needle, have the client verify the medication amount. ____ ____ ____ _____

17. Instruct client on procedure for mixing two medications in one syringe, if necessary. Discuss how much medication should be in the syringe at the end of the procedure. ____ ____ ____ _____

18. Instruct client to put cap or sheath back over needle without touching it. ____ ____ ____ _____

19. Show client sites for injection. Discuss rotation of sites. Assist client to select a site and wipe it with alcohol. ____ ____ ____ _____

20. When alcohol is dry, have client remove cap and show client how to hold syringe like a dart or pencil. ____ ____ ____ _____

21. For a SC injection, have client grasp or pinch injection site between thumb and forefingers of free hand. For the posterior upper arm, have client press back of arm against wall or chair and have client "roll" arm down to push up the skin. For an IM injection, have client hold the skin taut. ____ ____ ____ _____

22. Teach client to use a quick jab and insert the needle all of the way to the hub using the correct angle of insertion. ____ ____ ____ _____

23. Instruct client to let go of skin after needle is inserted and transfer free hand to barrel of syringe. ____ ____ ____ _____

24. For IM injection, explain the importance of aspirating before injecting the medication. Discuss how to aspirate and what to do if blood return is noted. ____ ____ ____ _____

25. Have client push plunger all of the way in a slow and steady rate to administer the medication. ____ ____ ____ _____

26. Teach client to pull needle straight out quickly after medication is administered. A small gauze pad may be held over the site after needle is removed. ____ ____ ____ _____

27. Teach client appropriate disposal of syringe. ____ ____ ____ _____

	S	U	NP	Comments

28. Explain safe reuse of needles for client with adequate immune system.

    _____ _____ _____ _____

29. Have client indicate on record chart where injection was given.

    _____ _____ _____ _____

30. Encourage client to ask questions about procedure and provide client with written and visual guidelines.

    _____ _____ _____ _____

31. Give client a bottle of sterile saline to practice preparing medication.

    _____ _____ _____ _____

Performance Checklist: Skill 18.2

Intramuscular Injections

	S	U	NP	Comments

Assessment

1. Review physician's orders for client's name, drug name, dose, time, and route of administration.

2. Gather information pertinent to drug(s) ordered.

3. Check expiration date of medication.

4. Consider factors that may contraindicate IM injection.

5. Assess client's medical history, history of allergies, and medication history.

6. Assess client's knowledge regarding medication and dosage schedule.

7. Observe client's verbal and nonverbal responses toward receiving injection.

Implementation

1. Use Standard Protocol.

Nurse Alert: Review the six "rights" of medication administration.

2. Prepare medication in syringe.

3. Identify client.

4. Explain procedure, location of injection site, and how positioning lessens discomfort. Proceed in calm manner.

5. Choose appropriate IM injection site (ventrogluteal preferred) by assessing size and integrity of muscle.

6. Assist client to comfortable position, depending on site.

7. Apply gloves. Relocate site using anatomical landmarks.

8. Carefully remove cap or sheath from needle.

9. With nondominant hand, pull the skin

1 to 1½ inches (2.5-3.5 cm) laterally down
so as to administer the injection in a
Z-track manner. Hold the skin taut.

_____ _____ _____ _____

10. Cleanse site with an antiseptic swab,
beginning at the center of the site and
moving outward in a circular direction for
about 2 inches (5 cm). Allow alcohol to dry.

_____ _____ _____ _____

11. Hold swab or gauze square between fingers
of nondominant hand or place near site.

_____ _____ _____ _____

12. Hold syringe between thumb and forefinger
of dominant hand as if holding a dart, with
palm down at 90-degree angle to client's skin.

_____ _____ _____ _____

13. Insert needle quickly. Aspirate for at least
5 to 10 seconds. Inject medication slowly
at a rate of 1 ml every 10 seconds.

_____ _____ _____ _____

**Nurse Alert: If blood appears, remove needle and
dispose of medication and syringe. Repeat
preparation procedure.**

14. Wait 10 seconds after injecting the
medication before withdrawing the needle.

_____ _____ _____ _____

15. Smoothly and steadily withdraw the
needle and release the skin. Apply gentle
pressure at site with dry sponge or swab.

_____ _____ _____ _____

16. Place small adhesive bandage if bleeding is
noted.

_____ _____ _____ _____

17. Discard sheathed or uncapped needle and
attached syringe into appropriate receptacle
using needle stick prevention techniques.
Discard gloves and wash hands.

_____ _____ _____ _____

18. Use Completion Protocol.

_____ _____ _____ _____

Evaluation

1. Observe for effects of prescribed IM
medication within 30 to 60 minutes.

_____ _____ _____ _____

2. Assess the injection site 2 to 4 hours after
injection for redness, swelling, pain, or
other effects.

_____ _____ _____ _____

3. Have client verbalize effect and purpose of
medication.

_____ _____ _____ _____

• Identify unexpected outcomes and
intervene as necessary.

_____ _____ _____ _____

• Record and report intervention and client's
response.

_____ _____ _____ _____

Performance Checklist: Skill 18.3

Intradermal Injections

	S	U	NP	Comments

Assessment

1. Review physician's orders for client's name, drug name, dose, time, and route of administration.

2. Gather information regarding drug(s) ordered.

3. Assess client's history of allergies, substance to which client is allergic, and normal allergic reaction.

4. Determine whether client has had previous reaction to skin testing.

5. Check date of expiration for medication vial or ampule.

6. Assess client's knowledge of purpose and reactions to skin testing.

Implementation

1. Use Standard Protocol.

Nurse Alert: Review the six "rights" of medication administration.

2. Prepare medication in syringe.

3. Identify client.

4. Select appropriate injection site: Avoid bruises and areas of inflammation, edema, lesions, or discoloration.

5. Assist client to comfortable position with elbow and forearm extended and supported on flat surface.

6. Apply gloves. Cleanse site with an antiseptic swab beginning at center of the site and rotating outward in a circular direction for about 2 inches (5 cm). Allow to dry.

7. Hold swab or square of sterile gauze between fingers of nondominant hand.

	S	U	NP	Comments

8. Remove needle cap or sheath from needle by pulling it straight off.

____ ____ ____ _____

9. Hold syringe between thumb and forefinger of dominant hand with bevel of needle pointing up.

____ ____ ____ _____

10. With nondominant hand, stretch skin over site with forefinger or thumb.

____ ____ ____ _____

11. With needle almost against client's skin, insert it carefully at a 5- to 15-degree angle until resistance is felt, and advance needle through epidermis to approximately ⅛ inch (3 mm) below skin surface. Needle tip can be seen through skin.

____ ____ ____ _____

12. Inject medication slowly. It is not necessary to aspirate. Normally, resistance is felt. If not, needle is too deep; remove and begin again.

____ ____ ____ _____

13. While injecting medication, a light-colored bleb resembling a mosquito bite approximately ¼ inch (6 mm) in diameter forms at site and gradually disappears.

____ ____ ____ _____

14. Withdraw needle while applying alcohol swab or gauze gently over site.

____ ____ ____ _____

15. Do not massage site.

____ ____ ____ _____

16. Discard uncapped needle and syringe in appropriately labeled receptacle.

____ ____ ____ _____

17. Read site within appropriate amount of time.

18. Use Completion Protocol.

____ ____ ____ _____

Evaluation

1. Evaluate for desired effect. Assess site of skin testing for erythema and induration.

____ ____ ____ _____

2. Assess for pain and any allergic symptoms.

____ ____ ____ _____

3. Inspect bleb. Use skin pencil and draw circle around perimeter of injection site. Tell client not to wash off markings.

____ ____ ____ _____

4. Ask client to describe implications of skin testing and expected reaction.

____ ____ ____ _____

• Identify unexpected outcomes and intervene as necessary.

____ ____ ____ _____

• Record and report intervention and client's response.

____ ____ ____ _____

Performance Checklist: Skill 18.4

Continuous Subcutaneous Medications

	S	U	NP	Comments

Assessment

1. Review physician's orders for client's name, drug name, dose, time, and route of administration.   ____ ____ ____ _____

2. Gather information regarding drug(s) ordered.   ____ ____ ____ _____

3. Check expiration date of medication.   ____ ____ ____ _____

4. Assess for factors that may contraindicate CSQI.   ____ ____ ____ _____

5. Assess client's medical history, history of allergies, and medication history.   ____ ____ ____ _____

6. Assess adequacy of client's adipose tissue to determine site.   ____ ____ ____ _____

7. Assess client's knowledge of medication and use of pump.   ____ ____ ____ _____

Implementation

1. Use Standard Protocol.

Nurse Alert: Review the six "rights" of medication administration.

2. To initiate CSQI:
   a. Prepare correct medication dose and prime tubing following manufacturer's directions.   ____ ____ ____ _____
   b. Obtain and program medication administration pump.   ____ ____ ____ _____
   c. Identify client.   ____ ____ ____ _____
   d. Explain procedure to client and proceed in a calm, confident manner.   ____ ____ ____ _____
   e. Select appropriate injection site.   ____ ____ ____ _____
   f. Assist client to a comfortable position.   ____ ____ ____ _____
   g. Apply gloves. Cleanse injection site with alcohol followed by povidone-iodine moving in a circular motion. Allow the alcohol and povidone-iodine to dry thoroughly.   ____ ____ ____ _____

Nurse Alert: Clients allergic to povidone-iodine may use an antibacterial soap to cleanse the site.

   h. Apply gloves. Hold needle in dominant hand and remove needle guard.   ____ ____ ____ _____

   i. With nondominant hand, pinch or lift

	S	U	NP	Comments

up the skin. Gently and firmly insert the needle at a 45- to 90-degree angle.

Nurse Alert: Some prepackaged needles are inserted at a 90-degree angle. Refer to maufacturer's directions.

    j. Release skinfold and apply tape over "wings" of needle.

Nurse Alert: Some cannulas have a sharp needle with a plastic catheter covering the needle. In this case, remove the needle and leave the plastic catheter in the skin.

    k. Place occlusive, transparent dressing over the insertion site.

    l. Attach tubing from needle to tubing from infusion pump and turn pump on.

Nurse Alert: Some pumps require additional priming at this point to clear air from the new infusion set. Refer to the pump manufacturer's instructions.

    m. Dispose of any sharps into appropriate receptacle. Discard gloves and wash hands.

    n. Assess site before leaving client and instruct client to inform nurse if site becomes red or begins to leak.

3. To discontinue CSQI:
    a. Verify order and establish alternative method for medication administration.
    b. Stop infusion pump.
    c. Apply gloves and remove dressing without dislodging needle.
    d. Cleanse site with alcohol followed by povidone-iodine if site is infected or according to agency policy.
    e. Remove tape from wings of needle or and pull needle out at the same cannula angle it was inserted.
    f. Apply gentle pressure at site until no fluid leaks out of skin.
    g. Apply small sterile gauze dressing or adhesive bandage to site.
    h. Discard used supplies and wash hands.

4. Use Completion Protocol.

Evaluation

1. Assess site at least every 4 hours.

2. Evaluate client's response to medication.

3. Ask client to describe medication and CSQI therapy.

- Identify unexpected outcomes and intervene as necessary.

- Record and report intervention and client's response.

Performance Checklist: Skill 19.1

Preoperative Assessment

	S	U	NP	Comments

Assessment and Implementation

1. Use Standard Protocol.

2. Determine whether the client has any communication impairment and if the client is mentally competent.

3. Assess the client's understanding of the intended surgery and anesthesia.

4. Obtain a nursing history.
   a. Condition leading to surgery
   b. Chronic illnesses
   c. Last menstrual period (for female clients in childbearing years)
   d. Previous hospitalizations
   e. Medication history, including prescription and over-the-counter (OTC), and date and time of last doses
   f. Previous experience with surgery and anesthesia
   g. Family history of complications from surgery or anesthesia
   h. Allergies to medications, foods, including specific questions about natural rubber latex
   i. Physical impairment
   j. Prostheses and implants (e.g., dentures, hearing aid, pacemaker, internal defibrillator, hip prosthesis)
   k. Smoking, alcohol, and drug use
   l. Occupation

5. Assess client's weight, height, and vital signs.

6. Assess client's respiratory status, including character and rate of respirations, oxygen saturation, ability to breathe lying flat, and chest x-ray report.

7. Assess client's circulatory status, including apical pulse, electrocardiogram (ECG) report, and peripheral pulses.

8. Determine client's neurological status, including level of consciousness (LOC).

	S	U	NP	Comments

9. Assess client's musculoskeletal system, including range of motion (ROM) of joints. ___ ___ ___ _____

10. Examine client's skin; identify any breaks in skin integrity and determine level of hydration. ___ ___ ___ _____

11. Assess client's emotional status, including level of anxiety, coping ability, and family support. ___ ___ ___ _____

12. Review the results of laboratory tests, including complete blood count (CBC), electrolytes, urinalysis, and other diagnostic tests. ___ ___ ___ _____

13. Ask if client has an advanced directive. ___ ___ ___ _____

14. Identify the time of client's last intake of food or drink. ___ ___ ___ _____

15. Use Completion Protocol. ___ ___ ___ _____

Evaluation

1. Review records to determine whether necessary information has been assessed. ___ ___ ___ _____

2. Evaluate client's ability to cooperate. ___ ___ ___ _____

- Identify unexpected outcomes and intervene as necessary. ___ ___ ___ _____

- Record and report intervention and client's response. ___ ___ ___ _____

Performance Checklist: Skill 19.2

Preoperative Teaching

	S	U	NP	Comments

Assessment

1. Ask about client's previous experiences with surgery and anesthesia. ___ ___ ___ _____

2. Determine client's and family's understanding of surgery. ___ ___ ___ _____

3. Identify client's cognitive level, language, and culture. ___ ___ ___ _____

4. Assess client's anxiety related to surgery. ___ ___ ___ _____

Implementation

1. Use Standard Protocol. ___ ___ ___ _____

2. Inform client and family of date, time, location of surgery, and where to wait. Inform client and family about the anticipated length of time of surgery. ___ ___ ___ _____

3. Answer questions client and family ask. ___ ___ ___ _____

4. Describe perioperative routines. ___ ___ ___ _____

5. Describe preoperative medications. ___ ___ ___ _____

6. Review which routine medications are to be discontinued before surgery. ___ ___ ___ _____

7. Describe perioperative sensations to expect (sights, sounds, touch). ___ ___ ___ _____

8. Describe pain control methods. Many clients have a patient-controlled analgesia (PCA) pump. ___ ___ ___ _____

9. Describe what client will experience postoperatively. ___ ___ ___ _____

10. Have client practice splinting. Hold pillow to abdomen for support while sitting up or coughing. ___ ___ ___ _____

11. Have client practice turning and sitting up.
    a. Flex knees while supine. ___ ___ ___ _____
    b. Splint incision with arm and pillow to turn to either side. ___ ___ ___ _____
    c. While splinting incision with arm, use free arm to grab side rail and turn onto side. ___ ___ ___ _____

d. To sit up on right side, turn onto right side. Push on the mattress with right arm and swing feet over the edge of the bed.   _____ _____ _____ _____

12. Have client practice deep breathing and coughing.
    a. Assist client to sitting position.   _____ _____ _____ _____
    b. Instruct client to place palms of hands over the lower border of the rib cage with third fingers touching.   _____ _____ _____ _____
    c. Have client take slow, deep breaths and feel fingers separate.   _____ _____ _____ _____
    d. Have client hold the breath for 3 seconds and exhale through the mouth slowly, as if blowing out a candle.   _____ _____ _____ _____
    e. Splint abdomen with pillow.   _____ _____ _____ _____
    f. Instruct client to cough forcefully after 4 to 6 deep breaths.   _____ _____ _____ _____
    g. Have client practice several times.   _____ _____ _____ _____
    h. Have client perform turn, cough, and deep breathing every 2 hours.   _____ _____ _____ _____

13. Instruct client in use of incentive spirometer.
    a. Position in a sitting or reclining position.   _____ _____ _____ _____
    b. Instruct client to exhale completely, then place mouthpiece so that lips completely cover it and inhale slowly, maintaining constant flow through unit.   _____ _____ _____ _____
    c. After maximum inspiration, client should hold breath for 2 to 3 seconds, then exhale slowly.   _____ _____ _____ _____
    d. Set marker on spirometer at maximum inspiration point.   _____ _____ _____ _____
    e. Instruct client to breathe normally for a short period, then repeat process.   _____ _____ _____ _____

14. Have client practice leg exercises.
    a. Position client supine.
    b. Rotate each ankle in a complete circle.   _____ _____ _____ _____
    c. Draw imaginary circles with the big toe five times.   _____ _____ _____ _____
    d. Alternate dorsiflexion and plantar flexion while instructing client to feel calf muscles tighten and relax. Repeat five times.   _____ _____ _____ _____
    e. Instruct client to alternate flexing and extending knees one leg at a time. Repeat five times.   _____ _____ _____ _____
    f. Instruct client to alternate straight leg raises. Repeat five times.   _____ _____ _____ _____
    g. Instruct client to perform these leg exercises 10 to 12 times every 2 hours while awake.   _____ _____ _____ _____

	S	U	NP	Comments

15. Verify that client's expectations of surgery are realistic. Correct expectations as needed. ____ ____ ____ _____

16. Reinforce therapeutic coping strategies. If ineffective, encourage alternatives. ____ ____ ____ _____

17. Use Completion Protocol. ____ ____ ____ _____

Evaluation

1. Ask client to repeat key information. ____ ____ ____ _____

2. Ask client to demonstrate splinting, turning and sitting, deep breathing, and leg exercises. ____ ____ ____ _____

3. Ask family to identify location of waiting room. ____ ____ ____ _____

4. Determine family's readiness to care for client after discharge. ____ ____ ____ _____

5. Observe emotional support provided by family.

6. Observe client and family coping strategies. ____ ____ ____ _____

- Identify unexpected outcomes and intervene as necessary. ____ ____ ____ _____

- Record and report intervention and client's response. ____ ____ ____ _____

Performance Checklist: Skill 19.3

Physical Preparations

	S	U	NP	Comments

Assessment and Implementation

1. Use Standard Protocol.

2. Assist client to put on hospital gown and remove personal items.

3. Instruct client to remove makeup, nail polish, hairpins, and jewelry.

4. Ensure that money and valuables have been locked up or given to a family member.

5. Verify that client's identification and blood band are correct and legible.

6. Ensure that client has had nothing to eat or drink during the past 8 hours.

7. Verify that client has taken medications as instructed.

8. Verify that a bowel preparation has been completed if ordered.

9. Ensure that a medical history and physical examination results are in client's record.

10. Verify that surgical consent is complete.

11. Ensure that necessary laboratory work, ECG, and chest x-ray studies have been completed.

12. Check that type and crossmatch has been completed if ordered by the physician and that blood transfusions are available as needed.

13. Ask if client has an advanced directive. If so, place it in client's record.

14. Assess and record client's heart rate, blood pressure, respiratory rate, oxygen saturation, and temperature.

15. Administer purgatives or enemas if ordered.

16. Instruct client to void.

17. Start an IV line; refer to unit standards or physician's orders.

18. Administer preoperative medications as ordered.
    —— —— —— ————————

Nurse Alert: Preoperative antibiotics should be administered within 2 hours preoperatively.

19. Apply antiembolism stockings.
    a. Measure client while standing, from gluteal fold to the floor, circumference of largest part of calf (refer to agency policy).
    —— —— —— ————————
    b. With the client lying down, invert the stocking and slip it over the foot.
    —— —— —— ————————
    c. Ease the stocking snugly over the leg.
    —— —— —— ————————

20. Apply sequential compression stockings if ordered.
    a. Measure around the largest part of the thigh.
    —— —— —— ————————
    b. Wrap stockings around the leg, starting at the ankle, with the opening over the patella.
    —— —— —— ————————
    c. Attach the stockings to the insufflator, and verify that the intermittent pressure is between 35 and 45 mm Hg.
    —— —— —— ————————

21. Cleanse and prepare the surgical site, if ordered.
    —— —— —— ————————

22. Insert a urinary catheter if ordered.
    —— —— —— ————————

23. Administer an enema, if ordered.
    —— —— —— ————————

24. Remove contact lenses, eyeglasses, hairpieces, and dentures.
    —— —— —— ————————

25. Place a cap on client's head.
    —— —— —— ————————

26. Assist client onto stretcher for transport to operating room.
    —— —— —— ————————

27. Use Completion Protocol.
    —— —— —— ————————

Evaluation

1. Evaluate client's ability to participate in preparation for surgery.
    —— —— —— ————————

2. Evaluate measures to reduce risk of infection.
    —— —— —— ————————

• Identify unexpected outcomes and intervene as necessary.
    —— —— —— ————————

• Record and report intervention and client's response.
    —— —— —— ————————

Performance Checklist: Skill 20.1

Surgical Hand Antisepsis

	S	U	NP	Comments

Assessment

1. Determine type and length of time for hand wash or scrub (check agency policy). _____ _____ _____ _____

2. Remove bracelets, rings, and watches. _____ _____ _____ _____

3. Inspect fingernails, which must be short, clean, and healthy. Remove artificial nails. _____ _____ _____ _____

4. Inspect skin and cuticles of hands and arms for abrasions, cuts, or open lesions. _____ _____ _____ _____

Implementation

1. Put on surgical shoe covers, cap or hood, face mask, and protective eyewear. _____ _____ _____ _____

2. Turn water on using foot or knee control and adjust to comfortable temperature. _____ _____ _____ _____

3. Wet hands and arms, keeping arms flexed with hands pointed upward, allowing the water to flow off at the elbows. _____ _____ _____ _____

4. Rinse hands and arms, keeping arms flexed with hands pointed upward, allowing the water to flow off at the elbows. _____ _____ _____ _____

5. Clean under nails of both hands with file under running water, then discard file. _____ _____ _____ _____

6. Surgical hand scrub (with brush)
   a. Wet brush and apply antimicrobial agent. Scrub the nails of one hand with 15 strokes. Scrub the palm, each side of thumb and fingers, and the posterior side of the hand with 10 strokes each. _____ _____ _____ _____
   b. Mentally divide the arm into thirds and scrub each third 10 times. Rinse brush and repeat sequence on other arm. _____ _____ _____ _____
   c. Discard brush; flex arms and rinse from fingertips to elbows in one continuous motion, allowing water to run off at elbow. _____ _____ _____ _____
   d. Turn off water with foot or knee control and back into room with hands elevated in from and away from body. _____ _____ _____ _____

e. Go to sterile setup and grasp sterile towel, taking care not to drip water on the sterile field.

    —— —— —— ———————

f. Bending slightly at the waist, use a sterile towel to dry one hand thoroughly, moving from fingers to elbow in a rotating motion.

    —— —— —— ———————

g. Transfer sterile towel to opposite end and repeat step e. for other hand.

    —— —— —— ———————

h. Drop towel into linen hamper or into circulating nurse's hands.

    —— —— —— ———————

7. Option: Antiseptic anatomic scrub (brushless)

a. Dispense 2 ml of antimicrobial agent into palm of one hand. Dip fingertips of opposite hand into prep and work under nails. Spread remaining hand prep over hand and up to just above elbow.

    —— —— —— ———————

b. Using another 2 ml of hand prep, repeat procedure with other hand.

    —— —— —— ———————

c. Dispense another 2 ml of hand prep into either hand and reapply to all aspects of both hands up to wrists. Allow to dry before applying gloves.

    —— —— —— ———————

Evaluation

1. Evaluate postoperative client for signs of surgical wound infection.

    —— —— —— ———————

•   Identify unexpected outcomes and intervene as necessary.

    —— —— —— ———————

Performance Checklist: Skill 20.2

Donning Sterile Gown and Closed Gloving

	S	U	NP	Comments

Assessment

1. Select proper size and type of sterile gloves.
   _____ _____ _____ _____

2. Select proper size and type of sterile surgical gown.
   _____ _____ _____ _____

Implementation

1. Open sterile gown and glove package on a clean, dry, flat surface.
   _____ _____ _____ _____

2. Perform surgical hand scrub.
   _____ _____ _____ _____

3. After drying hands, pick up gown (folded inside out) from sterile package, grasping the inside surface of gown at the collar.
   _____ _____ _____ _____

4. Lift folded gown directly upward and away from the table.
   _____ _____ _____ _____

5. Locate neckband; with both hands, grasp the inside front of gown just below neckline.
   _____ _____ _____ _____

6. Allow gown to open, keeping at arm's length away from body with the inside of gown toward body. Do not touch outside of gown or allow it to touch the floor.
   _____ _____ _____ _____

7. Slip both arms into armholes simultaneously (do not allow hands to move through cuff opening), keeping hands at shoulder level. Have circulating nurse pull on gown by reaching inside arm seams. Gown is pulled on, leaving sleeves covering hands.
   _____ _____ _____ _____

8. Have circulating nurse tie gown at neck and waist. If wraparound gown, sterile flap is not touched until sterile gloves have been applied.
   _____ _____ _____ _____

9. Apply gloves using the closed-glove method.
   a. With hands covered by gown cuffs and sleeves, open inner sterile glove package.
   _____ _____ _____ _____
   b. Grasp folded cuff of glove for dominant hand with nondominant hand.
   _____ _____ _____ _____
   c. Extend dominant forearm forward with palm up, and place palm of glove against

palm of dominant hand. Gloved fingers point toward elbow.

d. Grasp cuff edges with thumb and forefingers of dominant hand. Grasp back of glove cuff with nondominant hand. Extend fingers into glove and pull glove over cuff.

e. Grasp top of glove and underlying gown sleeve with covered nondominant hand. Extend fingers into glove, being sure glove's cuff covers gown cuff.

f. Glove nondominant hand in same manner with gloved, dominant hand. Keep hand inside sleeve. Be sure fingers are fully extended into both gloves.

10. For wraparound gown:

a. Grasp sterile waist tie with gloved hands and untie.

b. Pass tie to another sterile team member, who stands still, or wrap tie in sterile towel and pass to circulating nurse. Keep gown tie in left hand.

c. Allowing margin of safety, turn to the left one half turn, covering back with extended gown flap. Retrieve tie only from team member, and secure both ties in place.

Evaluation

1. Evaluate postoperative client for signs of surgical wound infection.

• Identify unexpected outcomes and intervene as necessary.

• Record and report intervention and client's response.

Performance Checklist: Skill 21.1

Providing Immediate Postoperative Care in the Postanesthesia Care Unit

	S	U	NP	Comments

Assessment

1. Obtain report from circulating nurse and anesthesiologist or nurse anesthetist.

2. Review client's preexisting conditions during operative procedure, including baseline and intraoperative vital signs, blood or fluid loss, fluid replacement, type of anesthesia, airway, and surgical wound, including surgical drains.

3. Consider the effects of the client's type of surgery and anesthesia and restrictions to movement.

Implementation

1. Use Standard Protocol.

2. As client enters postanesthesia care unit (PACU), attach oxygen tubing to regulator and check IV flow rates.

3. Connect any drainage tubes to intermittent suction.

4. Attach monitoring devices.

5. Compare vital signs with client's preoperative baseline. Continue assessing vital signs at least every 5 to 15 minutes until stable.

6. Apply gloves. Maintain airway after general anesthesia.
   a. If client is supine, elevate head of bed slightly, support neck extension, and turn head to side unless contraindicated. Client may need to be reminded to breathe.

Nurse Alert: Always stay with sedated client until respirations are well established. Client with artificial airway may gag, vomit, become restless, or stop breathing.

   b. Suction artificial airway and oral cavity if secretions accumulate. Assist client to spit out oral airway as gag reflex returns.

   _____ _____ _____ _____

7. Call client by name in normal tone of voice. If there is no response, attempt to arouse client by touching or gently moving a body part. Explain that surgery is over and you are in the RR.

   _____ _____ _____ _____

8. Encourage client to cough and deep breathe every 15 minutes.

   _____ _____ _____ _____

9. Inspect color of nail beds and skin. Palpate skin temperature.

   _____ _____ _____ _____

10. Assess closely for potential cardiovascular and pulmonary complications of anesthesia.

   _____ _____ _____ _____

11. Monitor responses after epidural or spinal anesthesia.
   a. Monitor for hypotension, bradycardia, and nausea and vomiting.

   _____ _____ _____ _____

   b. Maintain adequate IV infusion.

   _____ _____ _____ _____

   c. Keep client flat or with head slightly elevated and maintain position.

   _____ _____ _____ _____

   d. Client is observed in PACU until movement returns in extremities.

   _____ _____ _____ _____

   e. Assess respiratory status, level of sensation, and mobility in lower extremities.

   _____ _____ _____ _____

Nurse Alert: In an emergency situation, document interventions and evaluation as reported to physician.

12. Monitor drainage.
   a. Apply gloves. Observe dressing and drains for any evidence of bright red blood. Look underneath client for any pooling of bloody drainage.

   _____ _____ _____ _____

   b. Inform physician of unexpected bloody drainage, and reinforce dressing as indicated. Monitor for decreased blood pressure and increased pulse.

   _____ _____ _____ _____

   c. Inspect condition and contents of any drainage tubes and collecting devices. Note character and volume of drainage.

   _____ _____ _____ _____

   d. Observe amount, color, and appearance of urine from indwelling Foley catheter (if present).

   _____ _____ _____ _____

   e. If nasogastric (NG) tube is present, assess drainage. If not draining, check placement and irrigate if necessary with normal saline.

   _____ _____ _____ _____

   f. Monitor IV fluid rates. Observe IV site for signs of infiltration.

   _____ _____ _____ _____

	S	U	NP	Comments

13. Promote comfort.
    a. Provide mouth care. ___ ___ ___ _____
    b. Provide a warm blanket or active rewarming therapy to promote warmth and minimize shivering. ___ ___ ___ _____
    c. Assist with position changes and provide supportive pillows. ___ ___ ___ _____

14. Assess pain as client awakens, including quality, severity, and location. ___ ___ ___ _____

15. Provide pain medication as ordered and when vital signs have stabilized. ___ ___ ___ _____

16. Explain client's condition to the client, and inform of plans for transfer to nursing division or discharge to home. ___ ___ ___ _____

17. When client's condition is stabilized, contact anesthesiologist to approve transfer to clinical unit or release to home. ___ ___ ___ _____

18. Before discharge to home from the ambulatory surgery unit (ASU), provide verbal and written instructions.
    a. Inform client of signs and symptoms of possible complications. ___ ___ ___ _____
    b. Do not drive for 24 hours. ___ ___ ___ _____
    c. Avoid important legal decisions for 24 hours. ___ ___ ___ _____
    d. Care for surgical site. ___ ___ ___ _____
    e. Provide activity restrictions. ___ ___ ___ _____
    f. Control pain. ___ ___ ___ _____
    g. Provide dietary modifications. ___ ___ ___ _____
    h. Plan for follow-up visit. ___ ___ ___ _____
    i. Clarify reasons to call the physician. ___ ___ ___ _____

19. Use Completion Protocol. ___ ___ ___ _____

Evaluation

1. Observe respirations and auscultate breath sounds. ___ ___ ___ _____

2. Compare vitals signs to client's baseline and expected values. ___ ___ ___ _____

3. Inspect dressings for drainage. ___ ___ ___ _____

4. Measure I&O. ___ ___ ___ _____

5. Assess pain level. ___ ___ ___ _____

6. Complete specific assessment related to type of surgery. ___ ___ ___ _____

• Identify unexpected outcomes and intervene as necessary. ___ ___ ___ _____

• Record and report intervention and client's response. ___ ___ ___ _____

Performance Checklist: Skill 21.2

Providing Comfort Measures During Early Postoperative Recovery

	S	U	NP	Comments

Assessment

1. Obtain phone report from nurse in PACU.

2. Assist with transfer and complete initial assessment. Review chart to identify type of surgery, preoperative medical risks, and baseline vital signs.

3. Review surgeon's postoperative orders.

Implementation

1. Use Standard Protocol.

Initial postoperative care

2. Prepare bed in high position (level with the stretcher), with sheet folded to side. Make room for a stretcher to be easily placed beside bed.

3. Assist transport staff to move client from stretcher to bed.

4. Attach any existing oxygen tubing, position IV fluids, check IV flow rate, and check drainage tubes.

5. Maintain airway. If client remains sleepy or lethargic, keep head extended and support in side-lying position.

6. Take vital signs and compare readings to those from recovery (PACU).

7. Apply gloves, as indicated. Encourage coughing and deep breathing.

8. If NG tube is present, check placement and connect to proper drainage device. Connect all drainage tubes to suction as indicated, and secure to prevent tension.

9. Assess client's surgical dressing for appearance and presence and character of drainage. Unless contraindicated, outline drainage along the edges with a pen and reassess in 1 hour for increase. If no dressing present, inspect condition of wound.

10. Assess client for bladder distention. If Foley catheter is present, check placement and be sure it is draining freely and properly secured. Check continuous bladder irrigations or suprapubic catheter for urinary drainage.

  _____ _____ _____ _____

11. Explain that voiding is expected within 8 hours postoperatively.

  _____ _____ _____ _____

12. Measure all sources of fluid intake and output. Remove and discard gloves. Wash hands.

  _____ _____ _____ _____

13. Describe the purpose of equipment and frequent observations to client and significant others.

  _____ _____ _____ _____

14. Position client for comfort, maintaining correct body alignment. Avoid tension on surgical wound site.

  _____ _____ _____ _____

15. Place call light within reach and raise side rail. Instruct client to call for assistance to get out of bed.

  _____ _____ _____ _____

16. Assess the need for pain medication based on client's level of discomfort and last time analgesic was given. PCA may be used for pain control.

  _____ _____ _____ _____

Continued postoperative care

17. Assess vital signs at least every 4 hours or as ordered.

  _____ _____ _____ _____

18. Provide oral care at least every 2 hours as needed. If permitted, offer ice chips.

  _____ _____ _____ _____

19. Encourage to turn, cough, and deep breathe at least every 2 hours.

  _____ _____ _____ _____

20. Encourage use of incentive spirometer.

  _____ _____ _____ _____

21. Promote ambulation and activity as ordered. Assess vital signs before and after activity to assess tolerance.

  _____ _____ _____ _____

22. Progress from clear liquids to regular diet as tolerated if nausea and vomiting do not occur.

  _____ _____ _____ _____

23. If possible, include client and family in decision making and answer questions as they arise.

  _____ _____ _____ _____

24. Provide opportunity for clients who must adjust to a change in body appearance or function to verbalize feelings.

  _____ _____ _____ _____

	S	U	NP	Comments

25. Discuss plans for discharge with client and caregivers, including wound care, medications, activity restrictions, and complications that warrant notifying the physician. Clarify follow-up appointments and encourage quick access to emergency telephone numbers. ____ ____ ____ _____

26. Use Completion Protocol. ____ ____ ____ _____

Evaluation

1. Auscultate breath sounds. ____ ____ ____ _____

2. Obtain vital signs. ____ ____ ____ _____

3. Ask client to describe pain (scale 1 to 10) after moderate activity. ____ ____ ____ _____

4. Evaluate I&O records. ____ ____ ____ _____

5. Auscultate bowel sounds. ____ ____ ____ _____

6. Inspect incision. ____ ____ ____ _____

7. Ask client to describe ability to cope. ____ ____ ____ _____

8. Ask client to indicate signs and symptoms of complications that should be reported. ____ ____ ____ _____

9. Have client or caregiver describe postoperative care and plans for follow-up visit. ____ ____ ____ _____

• Identify unexpected outcomes and intervene as necessary. ____ ____ ____ _____

• Record and report intervention and client's response. ____ ____ ____ _____

Performance Checklist: Skill 22.1

Providing Surgical Wound Care

	S	U	NP	Comments

Assessment

1. Identify the wound's location, size (depth, length, width), type of incision, presence of drains and type of dressing. ____ ____ ____ _____

2. Review documentation related to healing of the incision, including approximation of wound edges and drainage from wound, to provide basis for comparison. ____ ____ ____ _____

3. Review culture reports to identify presence of pathogenic organisms. ____ ____ ____ _____

4. Assess client's comfort level and identify symptoms of anxiety. Administer prescribed analgesic 30 to 45 minutes before changing dressing if appropriate. ____ ____ ____ _____

5. Identify client's history of allergies. ____ ____ ____ _____

Implementation

1. Use Standard Protocol. ____ ____ ____ _____

2. Form cuff on waterproof bag and place it near bed. ____ ____ ____ _____

3. Apply gloves. Remove dressing, pulling tape toward suture line. ____ ____ ____ _____

4. Inspect dressing for drainage. Discard soiled dressings and gloves directly into appropriate receptacle. ____ ____ ____ _____

5. Assess incision for signs of healing. Describe appearance to client. Provide a mirror if needed and client wants to see incision. ____ ____ ____ _____

6. Open sterile supplies for dressing and antiseptic swabs using aseptic technique. Position for easy access without reaching over the sterile field. ____ ____ ____ _____

7. Put on sterile gloves. ____ ____ ____ _____

8. Cleanse the suture line from tip to bottom. Discard the antiseptic swab. ____ ____ ____ _____

	S	U	NP	Comments

9. Cleanse the skin along each side of the incision using a single, sterile antiseptic swab for each stroke.

10. To cleanse a drain site, use a circular stroke starting with the area immediately next to the drain and moving out from the drain.

11. Apply dry, sterile dressing and secure with tape with ends folded under 0.5 cm (¼ inch).

12. Use Completion Protocol.

Evaluation

1. Inspect incision with each dressing change.

2. Note appearance and amount of drainage.

3. Inspect skin integrity around drains.

4. Ask client to describe level of pain.

• Identify unexpected outcomes and intervene as necessary.

• Record and report intervention and client's response.

Performance Checklist: Skill 22.2

Monitoring and Measuring Drainage Devices

	S	U	NP	Comments

Assessment

1. Identify placement of closed wound drain or type of drainage system when client returns form surgery.

2. Inspect for tube patency by observing drainage movement through tubing in direction of the reservoir, and checking for intact connection sites.

Implementation

1. Use Standard Protocol.

2. Apply gloves. Empty Hemovac, VacuDrain, or Constavac.
   a. Open plug on port for emptying drainage reservoir, and slowly squeeze two flat surfaces together, tilting container in that direction.
   b. Drain contents into sterile measuring container.
   c. Place container on a flat surface and press downward until bottom and top are in contact.
   d. Hold surfaces together with one hand, cleanse opening with alcohol swab and plug with other hand, and immediately replace plug.
   e. Check for patency of drainage tubing and absence of tension on tubing.
   f. Note characteristics of drainage, measure volume. Remove and discard gloves and wash hands.

3. Empty Hemovac with wall suction.
   a. Turn suction off.
   b. Disconnect suction tubing from Hemovac port.
   c. Empty Hemovac.
   d. Attach tubing with graduated connector to open port and secure with tape.
   e. Set suction level as prescribed or on low if physician does not specify suction level.

4. Empty Jackson-Pratt drain.
   a. Open port on the end of bulb-shaped reservoir.

   _____ _____ _____   _____

   b. Hold bulb over drainage container to empty drainage. Compress bulb to reestablish vacuum. Cleanse ends of emptying port with alcohol sponge.

   _____ _____ _____   _____

   c. Compress bulb to re-establish vacuum. Replace cap immediately.

   _____ _____ _____   _____

   d. Note characteristics of drainage; measure volume and discard by flushing down the commode.

   _____ _____ _____   _____

   e. Proceed with inspection of skin and dressing change using drain sponges. Place the bulk of the dressings below the drain, depending on client's usual position.

   _____ _____ _____   _____

   f. Instruct client about anticipated postoperative drainage, expected progress of wound healing and drainage volume, and estimated date of removal of drain as volume diminishes.

   _____ _____ _____   _____

   g. Instruct client to keep drain lower than waist level when ambulating, sitting, and lying down.

   _____ _____ _____   _____

   h. Instruct client not to pull or tug on tubing; secure drain below incision to dressing with tape and safety pin.

   _____ _____ _____   _____

Nurse Alert: Be sure there is slack in the tubing from the reservoir to the wound.

5. Remove drains (Penrose, Jackson-Pratt, Hemovac).
   a. Check physician's order for drain removal.

   _____ _____ _____   _____

   b. Remove dressings, discard in receptacle, and clean the area around the drain.

   _____ _____ _____   _____

   c. If removing a Jackson-Pratt or Hemovac drain, release the suction on the drainage device by opening the drainage port.

   _____ _____ _____   _____

   d. Inform client that there will be a pulling sensation as the drain is removed.

   _____ _____ _____   _____

   e. Place a disposable drape adjacent to the area to receive the drain after removal.

   _____ _____ _____   _____

   f. Clip and remove the suture if present. Remove clean gloves and put on sterile gloves.

   _____ _____ _____   _____

   g. Grasp the drain with sterile forceps or sterile gloved fingers and gently remove the drain. Inform client that momentary increased tension is felt just before completion of the removal.

   _____ _____ _____   _____

   h. Immediately cover the stab wound with a 4 × 4 dressing.

   _____ _____ _____   _____

   i. Instruct client to notify you if dressing becomes saturated with drainage.

   _____ _____ _____   _____

	S	U	NP	Comments

6. Use Completion Protocol.   _____ _____ _____ _____

Evaluation

1. Empty container every 8 hours and sooner if half to two-thirds full. Compare amount and characteristics of drainage with what is expected to determine patency of tubing and functioning of drainage evacuator.   _____ _____ _____ _____

2. Inspect for drainage around wound that can indicate obstruction of drainage system.   _____ _____ _____ _____

3. Evaluate client's comfort level.   _____ _____ _____ _____

• Identify unexpected outcomes and intervene as necessary.   _____ _____ _____ _____

• Record and report intervention and client's response.   _____ _____ _____ _____

Performance Checklist: Skill 22.3

Removing Staples and Sutures (Including Applying Steri-Strips)

	S	U	NP	Comments

Assessment

1. Review physician's orders for specific directions related to suture or staple removal.

2. Check for allergies to antiseptic solutions or tape.

3. Assess client's level of comfort.

4. Inspect skin integrity of suture line for uniform closure of wound edges, normal color, and absence of drainage and inflammation.

Implementation

1. Use Standard Protocol.

2. Check to determine whether nurse may remove sutures.

3. Obtain supplies and prepare sterile field.

4. Apply gloves. Remove dressing and discard in proper receptacle. Remove gloves and dispose in same receptacle.

5. Inspect wound for approximation of wound edges and absence of drainage and inflammation.

6. Apply sterile gloves if required by policy.

7. Cleanse sutures or staples and healed incision with antiseptic swabs.

8. Remove staples.
   a. Place lower tips of staple remover under first staple.
   b. Squeeze handles together all the way (without lifting).
   c. When both ends of staple are visible, gently lift it away from skin surface. If necessary, alter the angle and remove one end at a time.
   d. Release handles of staple remover over container.
   e. Repeat steps for every other staple.

f. Palpate for healing ridge and approximation of incision edges before remaining staples are removed.

＿＿＿ ＿＿＿ ＿＿＿ ＿＿＿＿＿＿＿＿＿＿＿

9. Remove interrupted sutures.
   a. Hold scissors in dominant hand and forceps (clamp) in nondominant hand. Note position of indented tip of scissors.

   ＿＿＿ ＿＿＿ ＿＿＿ ＿＿＿＿＿＿＿＿＿＿＿

   b. Grasp knot of suture with forceps and gently pull while slipping tip of scissors under suture near skin.

   ＿＿＿ ＿＿＿ ＿＿＿ ＿＿＿＿＿＿＿＿＿＿＿

   c. Snip suture as close to skin as possible and pull the suture through from the other side.

   ＿＿＿ ＿＿＿ ＿＿＿ ＿＿＿＿＿＿＿＿＿＿＿

   d. Gently remove suture and place it on sterile gauze.

   ＿＿＿ ＿＿＿ ＿＿＿ ＿＿＿＿＿＿＿＿＿＿＿

   e. Repeat steps until every other suture has been removed.

   ＿＿＿ ＿＿＿ ＿＿＿ ＿＿＿＿＿＿＿＿＿＿＿

   f. Assess for healing ridge and approximation of incision edges before remaining sutures are removed.

   ＿＿＿ ＿＿＿ ＿＿＿ ＿＿＿＿＿＿＿＿＿＿＿

10. Remove continuous sutures.
    a. Snip suture close to skin surface at end distal to knot.

    ＿＿＿ ＿＿＿ ＿＿＿ ＿＿＿＿＿＿＿＿＿＿＿

    b. Snip second "suture" on same side.

    ＿＿＿ ＿＿＿ ＿＿＿ ＿＿＿＿＿＿＿＿＿＿＿

    c. Grasp knot and gently pull with continuous smooth action, removing suture from beneath the skin. Place suture on gauze.

    ＿＿＿ ＿＿＿ ＿＿＿ ＿＿＿＿＿＿＿＿＿＿＿

    d. Grasp and lift next suture, and snip with tip of scissors close to skin.

    ＿＿＿ ＿＿＿ ＿＿＿ ＿＿＿＿＿＿＿＿＿＿＿

    e. Grasp suture and gently remove loop of suture.

    ＿＿＿ ＿＿＿ ＿＿＿ ＿＿＿＿＿＿＿＿＿＿＿

    f. Repeat these steps until the end knot is reached. Cut the last one and remove it by grasping and pulling the knot.

    ＿＿＿ ＿＿＿ ＿＿＿ ＿＿＿＿＿＿＿＿＿＿＿

11. Remove blanket continuous suture.
    a. Cut the suture opposite the looped blanket edge.

    ＿＿＿ ＿＿＿ ＿＿＿ ＿＿＿＿＿＿＿＿＿＿＿

    b. Remove each "suture" by grasping at the looped end.

    ＿＿＿ ＿＿＿ ＿＿＿ ＿＿＿＿＿＿＿＿＿＿＿

12. Apply Steri-Strips.
    a. Gently cleanse suture line with antiseptic swab.

    ＿＿＿ ＿＿＿ ＿＿＿ ＿＿＿＿＿＿＿＿＿＿＿

    b. Using a strong light, carefully inspect incision to be sure all sutures are removed.

    ＿＿＿ ＿＿＿ ＿＿＿ ＿＿＿＿＿＿＿＿＿＿＿

    c. Apply tincture of benzoin to the skin on each side of suture line. Allow to dry.

    ＿＿＿ ＿＿＿ ＿＿＿ ＿＿＿＿＿＿＿＿＿＿＿

    d. Cut Steri-Strips to allow strips to extend 4 to 5 cm (1½-2 inches) on each side of the incision.

    ＿＿＿ ＿＿＿ ＿＿＿ ＿＿＿＿＿＿＿＿＿＿＿

    e. Remove backing and apply across incision.

    ＿＿＿ ＿＿＿ ＿＿＿ ＿＿＿＿＿＿＿＿＿＿＿

	S	U	NP	Comments

f. Apply light dressing if drainage is apparent or if clothing may rub and irritate the suture line, or the incision may be left.

_____ _____ _____ _____

g. Inform client to take showers rather than soak in bathtub according to physician's preference.

_____ _____ _____ _____

13. Review local and systemic indications of infection. Instruct client to notify physician if these occur after discharge.

_____ _____ _____ _____

14. Inform client to minimize abdominal strain during defecation and show how to support the incision with pillow or bath blanket.

_____ _____ _____ _____

15. Encourage ambulation.

_____ _____ _____ _____

16. Follow physician's instructions for limiting activity.

_____ _____ _____ _____

17. Provide written instructions as well as verbal instructions, allowing opportunity to answer questions as they arise.

_____ _____ _____ _____

18. Use Completion Protocol.

_____ _____ _____ _____

Evaluation

1. Inspect incision for approximation of wound edges.

_____ _____ _____ _____

2. Ask client to rate pain level.

_____ _____ _____ _____

3. Ask client to explain self-care guidelines.

• Identify unexpected outcomes and intervene as necessary.

_____ _____ _____ _____

• Record and report intervention and client's response.

_____ _____ _____ _____

Performance Checklist: Skill 23.1

Pressure Ulcer Risk Assessment and Prevention Strategies

	S	U	NP	Comments

Assessment

1. Select pressure ulcer risk assessment tool.

2. Identify client's risk for pressure ulcer formation by assessing the factors for each client according to the selected tool.

3. Assess condition of client's skin.

4. Assess client for additional areas of potential pressure.

5. Observe client for preferred positions when in bed or chair.

6. Observe ability of client to initiate and assist with position changes.

7. Assess client's and support person's understanding of risks for pressure ulcers and knowledge of skin care.

Implementation

1. Use Standard Protocol.

2. Inspect skin at least once a day.

3. Check all assistive devices for potential pressure points.

4. Evaluate client's pressure ulcer risk.

5. For immobility, inactivity, or poor sensory perception:
   a. Reposition client.
   b. Use 30-degree lateral position.
   c. Use pillow bridging when needed.
   d. Place client in bed on a pressure-reducing support surface.
   e. Place client in chair on a pressure-reducing surface and shift position at least once every hour.

6. Consider the following if friction and shear are risk factors.
   a. Use a turning sheet to reposition the client.

	S	U	NP	Comments

b. Moisturize areas that are prone to friction injuries. ____ ____ ____ _____

c. Maintain the head of the bed at 30 degrees. ____ ____ ____ _____

Nurse Alert: Do not massage reddened ares.

7. If the client receives a low score on the moisture subscale, consider one or more of the following:

a. Use a moisture barrier ointment after incontinent episodes. ____ ____ ____ _____

b. Use a protective barrier paste if skin is denuded. ____ ____ ____ _____

c. Consider a collection device if incontinence is ongoing. ____ ____ ____ _____

d. Perform frequent dressing changes and skin barriers for wound drainage. ____ ____ ____ _____

8. Consider the following if the client scores low on the nutrition subscale.

a. Assess client's nutritional status. ____ ____ ____ _____

b. Review weight pattern, serum albumin, and total lymphocyte values. ____ ____ ____ _____

c. Offer support with eating. ____ ____ ____ _____

d. Provide oral supplements, if necessary. ____ ____ ____ _____

e. Evaluate fluid intake. ____ ____ ____ _____

9. Provide education to client and support persons regarding pressure ulcer risk and prevention. ____ ____ ____ _____

10. Use Completion Protocol. ____ ____ ____ _____

Evaluation

1. Observe client's skin for areas at risk. ____ ____ ____ _____

2. Observe tolerance and ability of client to participate in position changes. ____ ____ ____ _____

3. Compare subsequent risk assessment scores and skin assessments. ____ ____ ____ _____

• Identify unexpected outcomes and intervene as necessary. ____ ____ ____ _____

• Record and report intervention and client's response. ____ ____ ____ _____

Performance Checklist: Skill 23.2

Treatment of Pressure Ulcers and Wound Management

	S	U	NP	Comments

Assessment

1. Assess client's level of comfort and need for pain management. ____ ____ ____ _____

2. Determine whether client has allergies to topical agents. ____ ____ ____ _____

3. Determine reason client has pressure ulcer to control or eliminate the cause. ____ ____ ____ _____

4. Review physician's order for topical agent or dressing. ____ ____ ____ _____

5. Assess each of the client's wounds and pressure ulcer(s) and surrounding skin to determine ulcer characteristics. ____ ____ ____ _____

6. Assess factors that affect wound healing. ____ ____ ____ _____

7. Assess nutritional status. ____ ____ ____ _____

8. Assess client's and support person's understanding of pressure ulcers and treatment. ____ ____ ____ _____

Implementation

1. Use Standard Protocol. ____ ____ ____ _____

2. Apply gloves. Select pressure ulcer management based on identified stage and other factors. ____ ____ ____ _____

3. Select an appropriate dressing based on assessment.
   a. Gauze pads ____ ____ ____ _____
   b. Transparent film ____ ____ ____ _____
   c. Hydrogel ____ ____ ____ _____
   d. Hydrocolloid ____ ____ ____ _____
   e. Alginate ____ ____ ____ _____
   f. Foam ____ ____ ____ _____

4. Open sterile packages and solution containers. ____ ____ ____ _____

5. Apply gloves. Arrange bed linen and client's gown to expose ulcer and surrounding skin. Keep remaining body parts draped. ____ ____ ____ _____

	S	U	NP	Comments

6. Remove old dressings and discard. Apply new gloves. ___ ___ ___ _____

7. Cleanse wound with prescribed solution.
   a. Rinse and dry skin surrounding ulcer. ___ ___ ___ _____
   b. Pulsed lavage may be used to loosen necrotic tissue. ___ ___ ___ _____
   c. Whirlpool treatments may be used to assist with wound debridement. ___ ___ ___ _____

8. Apply prescribed wound dressing.
   a. Gauze
      (1) Apply solution to gauze, then wring out. ___ ___ ___ _____
      (2) Unfold gauze and pack a deep wound or lay gauze over a shallow wound. ___ ___ ___ _____
      (3) Cover with a secondary dry dressing. ___ ___ ___ _____
   b. Transparent film dressing
   c. Hydrogel
      (1) Cover wound base with a thick layer of the amorphous hydrogel or cut a sheet to fit wound base. ___ ___ ___ _____
      (2) Cover with a secondary dressing and tape to secure in place. ___ ___ ___ _____
      (3) If using impregnated gauze, pack loosely into wound, cover with secondary dressing, and secure it in place. ___ ___ ___ _____
   d. Hydrocolloid
      (1) Select proper size, allowing at least 1 inch to extend beyond the wound edges. ___ ___ ___ _____
      (2) Remove paper backing from adhesive side and place over the wound. ___ ___ ___ _____
      (3) Hold in place for 30 to 60 seconds. ___ ___ ___ _____
   e. Alginate
      (1) Cut to the size of the wound and loosely pack into the wound. ___ ___ ___ _____
      (2) Cover with a secondary dressing and tape to secure in place. ___ ___ ___ _____
   f. Foam dressing
      (1) Select a dressing that extends 1 inch onto intact surrounding skin. ___ ___ ___ _____
      (2) Apply over wound and tape in place. ___ ___ ___ _____

9. Apply topical agents, as prescribed: antibacterials, antiseptics, enzyme debriding agents. ___ ___ ___ _____

10. Reposition client comfortably off wound. ___ ___ ___ _____

11. Use Completion Protocol. ___ ___ ___ _____

	S	U	NP	Comments

Evaluation

1. Evaluate condition of wound or ulcer and surrounding skin.

2. Inspect dressings and exposed wounds for evidence of drainage or tissue necrosis, odor, signs of systemic infection (fever and increased white blood cell count).

3. Compare periodic measurements.

4. Ask client to rate pain level.

• Identify unexpected outcomes and intervene as necessary.

• Record and report intervention and client's response.

Performance Checklist: Skill 24.1

Applying Dressings

	S	U	NP	Comments

Assessment

1. Assess size and location of wound to be dressed.

2. Ask client to rate pain using a scale of 0 to 10.

3. Assess client's knowledge of purpose of dressing change.

4. Determine the need for client or family member to participate in dressing wound.

Implementation

1. Use Standard Protocol.

2. Position client comfortably. Drape to expose only wound site. Instruct client not to touch wound or sterile supplies.

Nurse Alert:
Private room is indicated for clients with airborne, highly contagious infections.

Some dressings are reinforced rather than changed, such as postoperative dressings.

3. Place disposable waterproof bag within reach of work area with top folded to make a cuff.

4. Apply gloves. Remove tape: pull parallel to skin, toward dressing. If over hairy areas, remove in the direction of hair growth. Secure client permission to shave area (check agency policy).

5. With clean gloves, remove dressings one layer at a time observing appearance and drainage on dressing. Use caution to avoid tension on any drains that are present.

Nurse Alert: Moistening adherent dressings is no longer practiced.

6. Inspect wound for appearance, size, depth, drainage, integrity (wound edges are together), or granulation tissue.

7. Fold dressings with drainage contained inside and remove gloves inside out. (With small dressings, remove gloves inside out over dressing.) Dispose of gloves and soiled dressings in waterproof bag. Wash hands.

____ ____ ____ _____

8. Create sterile field with a sterile dressing tray or individually wrapped sterile supplies on overbed table. Pour prescribed solution into sterile basin.

____ ____ ____ _____

9. Use sterile gloves or no-touch technique with sterile forceps.

____ ____ ____ _____

10. Cleanse wound.
   a. Use a separate swab for each cleansing stroke.

   ____ ____ ____ _____

   b. Clean from least contaminated area to most contaminated.

   ____ ____ ____ _____

   c. Cleanse around drain (if present), using a circular stroke starting near the drain and moving outward.

   ____ ____ ____ _____

11. Use sterile, dry gauze to blot and dry wound.

____ ____ ____ _____

12. Apply antiseptic ointment if ordered, using same technique as for cleansing.

____ ____ ____ _____

13. Apply dressing.
   a. Apply dry, sterile dressing.
      (1) Apply loose, woven gauze as contact layer to promote proper absorption of drainage.

   ____ ____ ____ _____

      (2) Cut 4 × 4 gauze flat to fit around drain, if present. Precut gauze is also available.

   ____ ____ ____ _____

      (3) Apply second layer of gauze.

   ____ ____ ____ _____

      (4) Apply thicker woven pad.

   ____ ____ ____ _____

   b. Wet-to-dry dressing
      (1) Pour prescribed solution into sterile basin and add fine-mesh gauze.

   ____ ____ ____ _____

      (2) Apply moist fine-mesh gauze as a single layer directly onto wound surface. If wound is deep, gently pack gauze into wound with forceps until all wound surfaces are in contact with moist gauze.

   ____ ____ ____ _____

Nurse Alert: If wound is deep, gently lay gauze over wound surface with forceps until all surfaces are in contact with moist gauze and the wound is loosely filled. Avoid packing the wound too tightly.

      (3) Observe that dead space is loosely packed with gauze.
      (4) Apply dry, sterile 4 × 4 gauze over wet gauze.

   ____ ____ ____ _____

	S	U	NP	Comments

(5) Cover with ABD pad, Surgipad, or gauze. _____ _____ _____ _____

14. Secure dressing.
   a. Apply tape to secure dressing. _____ _____ _____ _____
   b. Montgomery ties
      (1) Expose adhesive surface of tape ends. A protective skin barrier is recommended. _____ _____ _____ _____
      (2) Place ties on opposite sides of the dressing. _____ _____ _____ _____
      (3) Secure dressing by lacing ties across dressing snugly enough to hold dressings secure but without pressure on the skin. _____ _____ _____ _____
   c. On an extremity, dressing is secured with roller gauze or Surgiflex elastic net. _____ _____ _____ _____

15. Remove cover gown and goggles. Remove gloves inside out and dispose of them in a waterproof container. Wash hands. _____ _____ _____ _____

16. Use Completion Protocol. _____ _____ _____ _____

Evaluation

1. Evaluate condition of wound. _____ _____ _____ _____

2. Ask client to rate pain level. _____ _____ _____ _____

3. Inspect status of dressing every shift and prn. _____ _____ _____ _____

4. Evaluate client/caregiver ability to perform dressing change. _____ _____ _____ _____

• Identify unexpected outcomes and intervene as necessary. _____ _____ _____ _____

• Record and report intervention and client's response. _____ _____ _____ _____

Performance Checklist: Skill 24.2

Changing Transparent Dressings

	S	U	NP	Comments

Assessment

1. Assess location, appearance, and size of wound to be dressed to allow nurse to determine supplies and assistance needed. ___ ___ ___ _____

2. Determine size of dressing needed. ___ ___ ___ _____

3. Assess pain level with pain scale. ___ ___ ___ _____

Implementation

1. Use Standard Protocol. ___ ___ ___ _____

2. Cuff top of disposable waterproof bag to prevent contamination of outer bag. Place within easy reach of work area. ___ ___ ___ _____

3. Apply gloves. Apply moisture-proof gown, mask, and goggles, if needed. Remove old dressing by pulling back slowly across dressing in direction of hair growth and toward the center. ___ ___ ___ _____

4. Remove disposable gloves by pulling them inside out over soiled dressings and dispose of them in waterproof bag. ___ ___ ___ _____

5. Prepare supplies. ___ ___ ___ _____

6. Reapply sterile (or clean) gloves if risk of exposure to body secretions is present. ___ ___ ___ _____

7. Cleanse area gently, swabbing toward area of most exudate, or spray with cleanser (check agency policy and physician preference). ___ ___ ___ _____

8. Dry skin around wound thoroughly with sterile gauze. ___ ___ ___ _____

9. Inspect wound for color, odor, and drainage; measure if indicated. ___ ___ ___ _____

10. Apply transparent dressing according to manufacturer's directions. ___ ___ ___ _____
    a. Remove paper backing, taking care not to allow adhesive areas to touch each other. ___ ___ ___ _____

	S	U	NP	Comments

b. Place film smoothly over wound without stretching.

c. Label with date, initials, and time if required by agency policy.

11. Remove gloves and discard in waterproof bag.

12. Use Completion Protocol.

Evaluation

1. Evaluate appearance of wound and compare with previous assessment.

2. Inspect condition of surrounding tissues.

3. Evaluate pain level.

• Identify unexpected outcomes and intervene as necessary.

• Record and report intervention and client's response.

Performance Checklist: Skill 24.3

Applying Binders and Bandages

	S	U	NP	Comments

Assessment

1. Observe client with need for support of thorax or abdomen. Observe ability to breathe deeply and cough effectively. _____ _____ _____ _____

2. Review medical record for order of binder type. _____ _____ _____ _____

3. Inspect skin for actual or potential alterations in integrity. _____ _____ _____ _____

4. Inspect surgical dressing. _____ _____ _____ _____

5. Assess client's comfort level, using a scale of 0 to 10 and noting any objective signs and symptoms. _____ _____ _____ _____

Implementation

1. Use Standard Protocol. _____ _____ _____ _____

Nurse Alert: Cover any exposed areas of wound or incision with sterile dressing.

2. Apply gloves, if needed. _____ _____ _____ _____

3. Apply binder.
   a. Abdominal binder
      (1) Position client in supine position with head slightly elevated and knees slightly flexed. _____ _____ _____ _____
      (2) Fanfold far side of binder toward midline of binder. _____ _____ _____ _____
      (3) Instruct and assist client to roll away from nurse toward raised side rail while firmly supporting abdominal incision and dressing with hands. _____ _____ _____ _____
      (4) Place fanfolded ends of binder under client. _____ _____ _____ _____
      (5) Instruct or assist client to roll over folded ends. _____ _____ _____ _____
      (6) Unfold and stretch ends out smoothly on far side of bed. _____ _____ _____ _____
      (7) Instruct client to roll back into supine position. _____ _____ _____ _____

S   U   NP   Comments

(8) Adjust binder so that supine client
     is centered over binder using
     symphysis pubis and costal margins
     as lower and upper landmarks.   ____ ____ ____ _____
(9) Close binder. Pull one end of binder
     over center of client's abdomen.
     While maintaining tension on that
     end of binder, pull opposite end
     of binder over center and secure
     with Velcro closure tabs, metal
     fasteners, or horizontally placed
     safety pins.   ____ ____ ____ _____
(10) Assess client's comfort level.   ____ ____ ____ _____
(11) Adjust binder as necessary.   ____ ____ ____ _____
b. Breast binder
  (1) Assist client in placing arms through
       binder's armholes.   ____ ____ ____ _____
  (2) Assist client to supine position in bed. ____ ____ ____ _____
  (3) Pad area under breasts if necessary.   ____ ____ ____ _____
  (4) Using Velcro closure tabs or
       horizontally placed safety pins,
       secure binder at nipple level first.
       Continue closure process above and
       then below nipple line until entire
       binder is closed.   ____ ____ ____ _____
  (5) Make appropriate adjustments,
       including individualizing fit of
       shoulder straps and pinning waistline
       darts to reduce binder size.   ____ ____ ____ _____
  (6) Instruct and observe skill development
       in self-care related to reapplying
       breast binder.   ____ ____ ____ _____

4. Remove and dispose of gloves, if worn.   ____ ____ ____ _____

5. Remove binder at scheduled intervals to
   assess underlying skin integrity (check
   agency policy).   ____ ____ ____ _____

6. Use Completion Protocol.   ____ ____ ____ _____

Evaluation

1. Evaluate pain level.   ____ ____ ____ _____

2. Observe client's respiratory status when
   using an abdominal or breast binder.   ____ ____ ____ _____

3. Observe site to be sure underlying dressings
   and skin are intact.   ____ ____ ____ _____

4. Remover binder and observe undelying skin. ____ ____ ____ _____

• Identify unexpected outcomes and
  intervene as necessary.   ____ ____ ____ _____

• Record and report intervention and client's
  response.   ____ ____ ____ _____

Performance Checklist: Skill 24.4

Wound Vacuum Assisted Closure

	S	U	NP	Comments

Assessment

1. Assess location and appearance of wound.

2. Ask client to rate pain using a scale of 0 to 10.

3. Assess client's knowledge of purpose of dressing change.

4. Determine the need for client or family member to participate in dressing wound.

Implementation

1. Use Standard Protocol.

2. Position client comfortably. Drape to expose only wound site. Instruct client not to touch wound or sterile supplies.

3. Place disposable waterproof bag within reach of work area with top folded to make a cuff.

4. Push therapy "on/off" button.
   a. Apply gloves. Keeping tube connectors with VAC unit, disconnect tubes from each other to drain fluids into canister.
   b. Prior to lowering, tighten clamp on canister tube.

5. With dressing tube unclamped, introduce 10 to 30 ml of normal saline, if ordered, into tubing to soak underneath foam.

6. Gently stretch transparent film horizontally and slowly pull up from the skin.

7. Remove old VAC dressing, observing appearance and drainage. Avoid tension on any drains that are present. Discard dressing and remove gloves.

Nurse Alert: If this is a new surgical wound, sterile technique may be ordered. Chronic wounds may use clean technique.

8. Apply sterile or clean gloves. Irrigate the wound with normal saline or other solution as ordered. Gently blot to dry.

9. Measure wound as ordered. Remove and discard gloves.

Nurse Alert: Wound cultures may be ordered on a routine basis or necessary based on assessment of wound.

10. Apply new sterile or clean gloves.

11. Prepare VAC foam.
    a. Select appropriate foam.
    b. Using sterile scissors, cut foam to wound size.

Nurse Alert: Clients may experience more discomfort with the black foam due to excessive wound contraction and may need to be switched to PVA soft-foam.

12. Gently place foam in wound, being sure that foam is in contact with entire wound base, margins, and undermined areas.

13. Apply tubing to foam in the wound.

Nurse Alert: If wound is deep, regularly reposition tubing to minimize pressure on wound edges. Reposition clients with restricted mobility and/or sensation frequently so they do not lie on tubing.

14. Apply skin protectant around the wound.

15. Cover the VAC foam, 3 to 5 cm of surrounding tissue, and tubing with wrinkle-free transparent film to ensure an occlusive seal. Do not apply tension to drape and tubing.

16. Secure tubing several centimeters away from the dressing.

17. Connect the tubing from the dressing to the tubing from the canister and VAC unit.
    a. Remove canister from sterile packaging and push into VAC unit until a click is heard. An alarm will sound if the canister is not properly engaged.
    b. Connect the dressing tubing to the canister tubing. Make sure both clamps are open.
    c. Place VAC unit on a level surface or hand from the foot of the bed. The unit will alarm and deactivate therapy if the unit is tilted beyond 45 degrees.
    d. Press in green-lit power button and set pressure as ordered.

	S	U	NP	Comments

18. Discard old dressing materials and remove gloves.

   ____ ____ ____ _____

19. Inspect wound VAC system to verify that negative pressure is achieved.
    a. Verify that display screen reads THERAPY ON.

   ____ ____ ____ _____

    b. Be sure that clamps are open and tubing is patent.

   ____ ____ ____ _____

    c. Identify air leaks by listening with stethoscope or by moving hand around edges of wound while applying light pressure.

   ____ ____ ____ _____

    d. Uses strips of transparent film to patch areas where there are leaks.

   ____ ____ ____ _____

20. Use Completion Protocol.

   ____ ____ ____ _____

Evaluation

1. Compare appearance of wound with prior assessment.

   ____ ____ ____ _____

2. Ask client to rate pain level.

   ____ ____ ____ _____

3. Verify airtight dressing seal and proper negative pressure.

   ____ ____ ____ _____

4. Evaluate client/caregiver ability to perform dressing change.

   ____ ____ ____ _____

- Identify unexpected outcomes and intervene as necessary.

   ____ ____ ____ _____

- Record and report intervention and client's response.

   ____ ____ ____ _____

Performance Checklist: Skill 25.1

Moist Heat

	S	U	NP	Comments

Assessment

1. Inspect wound dimensions and character, pain and drainage amount, color consistency, and odor.

2. Assess skin around wound and in area for integrity, color temperature, edema, pain, and sensitivity to touch.

3. Measure joint range of motion.

4. Assess client for altered perception of heat.

Implementation

1. Use Standard Protocol.

2. Provide warmth for client and position for comfort.

3. Place waterproof pad under area (except for sitz bath).

4. Apply moist compress.
   a. Clean moist compress to intact skin
      (1) Apply clean gloves for nonsterile compress. Heat prescribed solution to desired temperature.
      (2) Test solution temperature by placing small amount over forearm.
      (3) Pour solution into clean basin.
      (4) Place gauze or towel into solution.
      (5) Remove gauze or towel form basin.
   b. Sterile moist compress to open skin

Nurse Alert: Do not apply if bleeding, redness, inflammation, or fever is present.

      (1) Heat prescribed solution.
      (2) Test solution temperature by pouring small amount over back of hand. Solution should feel warm but not uncomfortably so.
      (3) Open package of sterile gauze and pour solution over gauze. Option: Place sterile gauze into basin and pour in solution.

	S	U	NP	Comments

    (4) Remove dressing, inspect wound, and dispose of dressing and gloves.

    (5) Put on sterile gloves.

    (6) Remove gauze from basin or waterproof package.

5. Wring excess moisture out of compress and place lightly on area.

6. Assess area for tolerance to application.

7. Cover with clean or sterile dry dressing and then dry bath towel.

8. Secure with tape or ties. Tell client to inform nurse if compress feels uncomfortably hot.

9. Repeat steps 1 to 8 every 5 minutes or as ordered.

10. Apply aquathermia pad over compress, if ordered.

Nurse Alert: Local application of heat greater than 20 minutes may result in vasoconstriction.

11. Provide warm soak to intact or open skin.
    a. Apply gloves. Cleanse intact skin or skin around open area with clean cloth and soap water or sterile gauze and sterile water.
    b. Pour heated solution into clean or sterile basin.
    c. Remove dressing and dispose of it and gloves.
    d. Immerse area into solution.
    e. Every 10 minutes, empty solution and replace with new.

12. Provide sitz bath to intact or open skin.
    a. Set sitz bath under toilet seat, hang bag above the level of the toilet seat, and connect tubing into sitz bath.
    b. Pour heated solution into bag after testing temperature of solution.
    c. Fill sitz bath one-third full of solution from the bag by opening the clamp on tubing.
    d. If there is a dressing, remove it and dispose of it and gloves.
    e. Assist client to sit in solution.
    f. Loosen clamp to regulate flow of warmed solution.
    g. Every 5 to 10 minutes, assess client for tolerance of treatment.

	S	U	NP	Comments

Nurse Alert: Hypotension can develop in clients with cardiac history. Monitor BP and dizziness or lightheadedness.

    h. Remove treatment after a total of 20 minutes. Sitz bath may be repeated after client has been out of the bath for 15 minutes.

  13. Use Completion Protocol.

Evaluation

1. Evaluate wound size, appearance, pain, and drainage.

2. Evaluate client's level of pain.

3. Inspect skin integrity around wound.

4. Measure joint range of motion.

• Identify unexpected outcomes and intervene as necessary.

• Record and report intervention and client's response.

Name _____ Date _____ Instructor's Name _____

Performance Checklist: Skill 25.2

Dry Heat

	S	U	NP	Comments

Assessment

1. Ask client to report pain level on scale of 0 to 10.

2. Assess range of motion of body part.

3. Assess client's skin for integrity, color, temperature, sensitivity to touch, blistering, and excessive dryness.

4. Check temperature level of external heating device to ensure function.

Implementation

1. Use Standard Protocol.

2. Prepare heat application.
   a. Aquathermia pad
      (1) Turn aquathermia unit on.

Nurse Alert: Setting exceeding 105° F should never be used. Avoid placing under a body part or positioning client directly on pad. Have client notify nurse if uncomfortably hot.

   (2) If uncovered, wrap with towel.
   b. Electric heating pad
      (1) Turn pad on. Set temperature to low or medium.
      (2) If uncovered, wrap pad with towel.
   c. Commercial heat pack

Nuse Alert: Do not puncture outer pack.

   (1) Break pouch inside larger pack.
   (2) Knead to mix chemicals.
   (3) Wrap pack in washcloth or soft cloth.

3. Place heat application on intact skin.

Nuse Alert: Never use pins to secure heating pads or packs.

4. Secure with cloth tape or ties.

5. Monitor condition of site every 5 minutes, assessing client's tolerance of treatment.

	S	U	NP	Comments

6. Remove treatment after 20 to 30 minutes (or time ordered by prescriber). ____ ____ ____ _____

7. Use Completion Protocol. ____ ____ ____ _____

Evaluation

1. Evaluate client's comfort level. ____ ____ ____ _____

2. Assess skin condition. ____ ____ ____ _____

3. Evaluate range of motion. ____ ____ ____ _____

4. Assess skin turgor to determine hydration. ____ ____ ____ _____

• Identify unexpected outcomes and intervene as necessary. ____ ____ ____ _____

• Record and report intervention and client's response. ____ ____ ____ _____

Performance Checklist: Skill 25.3

Cold Compresses and Ice Bags

	S	U	NP	Comments

Assessment

1. Assess client's pain on scale of 1 to 10.

2. Assess area or wound for edema and bleeding.

3. Assess surrounding skin for integrity, color, temperature, and sensitivity to touch.

Implementation

1. Use Standard Protocol.

2. Provide warm covering for client.

3. Position client carefully, keeping affected body part in proper alignment and exposing only the area to be treated.

Nurse Alert: Sterile supplies must be used with open wounds.

4. Prepare cold application.
   a. Cold compress. Apply gloves, as needed.
      (1) Place ice and water into basin.
      (2) Test temperature of solution.
      (3) Place gauze or towel into solution.
      (4) Wring excess solution from compress.
   b. Ice pack
      (1) Fill bag with water, then empty.
      (2) Fill bag two-thirds full with ice and water.
      (3) Express air from bag.
      (4) Secure closure. Wipe bag dry.
      (5) Place in second bag, if desired.
      (6) Wrap with towel or pillowcase.
   c. Commercial gel pack
      (1) Remove pack from freezer.
      (2) Wrap pack in towel or pillowcase.
      (3) Cover client's skin with towel.
   d. Electrical controlled or gravity cooling device
      (1) Make sure all connections are intact and temperature is set. (See agency policy, prescriber's order, and manufacturer's directions.)

	S	U	NP	Comments

(2) Cover cool water flow pad with towel. ___ ___ ___ _____

5. Apply cover device and apply cold
application to intact, protected skin. ___ ___ ___ _____

6. Secure with gauze, cloth tape, or ties. ___ ___ ___ _____

7. Remove treatment when the area feels numb
to the client. ___ ___ ___ _____

8. Use Completion Protocol. ___ ___ ___ _____

Evaluation

1. Evaluate client's pain level. ___ ___ ___ _____

2. Inspect tissue for edema, bruising, or
bleeding. ___ ___ ___ _____

3. Evaluate surrounding tissues for integrity,
color, temperature, and sensitivity to touch.
Repeat in 30 minutes. ___ ___ ___ _____

• Identify unexpected outcomes and
intervene as necessary. ___ ___ ___ _____

• Record and report intervention and client's
response. ___ ___ ___ _____

Performance Checklist: Skill 26.1

Using a Support Surface Overlay or Mattress

	S	U	NP	Comments

Assessment

1. Assess client's risk for pressure ulcer formation using a validated assessment tool. ____ ____ ____ _____

2. Perform skin assessment. ____ ____ ____ _____

3. Assess client's level of comfort and presence of pain. ____ ____ ____ _____

4. Assess client's understanding of purposes of support surfaces. ____ ____ ____ _____

5. Verify physician's order for surface. ____ ____ ____ _____

Implementation

1. Use Standard Protocol. ____ ____ ____ _____

2. Close room door or bedside curtain. ____ ____ ____ _____

3. Apply support surface to bed or prepare alternate bed (bed may be occupied or unoccupied). ____ ____ ____ _____
   a. Mattress replacement
      (1) Apply mattress to bed frame after removing standard hospital mattress. ____ ____ ____ _____
      (2) Apply sheet over mattress. ____ ____ ____ _____
   b. Air mattress/overlay
      (1) Apply deflated mattress flat over surface of bed mattress. (There may be directions on pad indicating which side to place up.) ____ ____ ____ _____

Nurse Alert: Avoid use of sharp objects near mattress.

   (2) Bring any plastic strips or flaps around corners of bed mattress. ____ ____ ____ _____
   (3) Attach connector on air mattress to inflation device. Inflate mattress to proper air pressure determined by air pump or blower. ____ ____ ____ _____
   (4) Place sheet over air mattress, being sure to eliminate all wrinkles. ____ ____ ____ _____
   (5) Check air pumps to be sure pressure cycle alternates. ____ ____ ____ _____

	S	U	NP	Comments

c. Air-surface bed
   (1) Obtain and make bed.   ____ ____ ____ _____
   (2) Place switch in the "Prevention" mode.   ____ ____ ____ _____

Nurse Alert: This and other support beds are equipped with a CPR switch to instantly lower the head and deflate the mattress.

4. Position client comfortably as desired over support surface. Reposition routinely.   ____ ____ ____ _____

5. Reassess the client's level of risk for skin breakdown and periodically verify the bed or mattress is still appropriate and necessary.   ____ ____ ____ _____

6. Instruct the client to call for assistance to get into and out of the bed.   ____ ____ ____ _____

7. Use Completion Protocol.   ____ ____ ____ _____

Evaluation

1. Evaluate skin condition every 8 hours.   ____ ____ ____ _____

2. Assess existing ulcers for evidence of healing.   ____ ____ ____ _____

3. Ask client to rate comfort level.   ____ ____ ____ _____

• Identify unexpected outcomes and intervene as necessary.   ____ ____ ____ _____

• Record and report intervention and client's response.   ____ ____ ____ _____

Performance Checklist: Skill 26.2

Using a Low-Air-Loss Bed

	S	U	NP	Comments

Assessment

1. Use a validated instrument to determine client's risk for pressure ulcer formation. ___ ___ ___ _____

2. Carefully inspect the skin for erythema, especially over bony prominences. ___ ___ ___ _____

3. Assess client's level of comfort and presence of pain. ___ ___ ___ _____

4. Assess client's understanding of the purposes of support surfaces. ___ ___ ___ _____

5. Review medical orders. ___ ___ ___ _____

Implementation

1. Use Standard Protocol. ___ ___ ___ _____

2. Close client's room door or bedside curtain. ___ ___ ___ _____

3. Explain steps of transfer. ___ ___ ___ _____

4. Transfer client to bed using appropriate transfer techniques. Turn bed on by depressing switch. Set Instaflate to allow safe and easy transfer. ___ ___ ___ _____

5. Release Instaflate and regulate temperature after transfer. ___ ___ ___ _____

6. Position client and perform range-of-motion exercises as appropriate. ___ ___ ___ _____

7. To turn clients, position bedpans, or perform other therapies, set Instaflate. Once procedure is completed, release Instaflate. ___ ___ ___ _____

Nurse Alert: CPR switch deflates bed quickly. Pressure relief is not received when bed is firm for procedures.

8. Identify special features required. Special features include:
   a. Scales for client weight ___ ___ ___ _____
   b. Portable transport units to maintain inflation when power source is interrupted ___ ___ ___ _____

	S	U	NP	Comments

c. Specialty cushions to allow patient positioning

d. Lateral rotation features that allow approximately 30 degrees of turning

9. Provide adequate fluid intake.

10. Use Completion Protocol.

Evaluation

1. Evaluate client's skin condition.

2. Inspect status of pressure ulcers.

3. Ask about level of comfort.

4. Observe LOC and orientation.

• Identify unexpected outcomes and intervene as necessary.

• Record and report intervention and client's response.

Performance Checklist: Skill 26.3

Using an Air-Fluidized Bed

	S	U	NP	Comments

Assessment

1. Use a validated risk assessment tool to determine client's risk for pressure ulcer formation. _____ _____ _____ _____

2. Carefully inspect the skin for evidence of pressure and impending breakdown. _____ _____ _____ _____

3. Review client's temperature and serum electrolytes. _____ _____ _____ _____

4. Assess client's emotional response and level of orientation. _____ _____ _____ _____

5. Identify clients at risk for complications of air-fluidized therapy. _____ _____ _____ _____

6. Review medical orders. _____ _____ _____ _____

Implementation

1. Use Standard Protocol. _____ _____ _____ _____

2. Review manufacturer's instructions. Premedicate client 30 minutes before transfer if needed. Obtain additional personnel for assistance. _____ _____ _____ _____

3. Transfer client onto air-fluidized bed using appropriate transfer techniques. _____ _____ _____ _____

4. Depress "on" switch to begin fluidization; regulate temperature. _____ _____ _____ _____

5. Position client and perform ROM exercises routinely. Foam wedges may be needed to place client in a Fowler's position. _____ _____ _____ _____

6. Use fluidization switch to harden bed for turning, positioning bedpans, and other procedures. Remember to reactivate fluidization after procedure. _____ _____ _____ _____

Nurse Alert: Activate CPR switch when resuscitation is necessary.

7. Obtain assistance when positioning client. _____ _____ _____ _____

8. Use a foam wedge to facilitate elevating the client's head for position changes. _____ _____ _____ _____

	S	U	NP	Comments

9. Inspect bony prominences and heels for signs of pressure every 8 to 12 hours. Avoid use of underpads.

    _____ _____ _____ _____

10. Apply gloves. Replace soiled sheets as needed, which are sent to the rental company for cleaning.

    _____ _____ _____ _____

11. Maintain adequate nutritional and fluid intake.

    _____ _____ _____ _____

12. Use Completion Protocol.

    _____ _____ _____ _____

Evaluation

1. Evaluate condition of skin periodically to determine changes in skin and effectiveness of air-fluidized therapy.

    _____ _____ _____ _____

2. Ask client to rate comfort level.

    _____ _____ _____ _____

3. Observe moisture of client's skin and mucous membranes and skin turgor. Monitor client's temperature and laboratory serum electrolytes.

    _____ _____ _____ _____

4. Evaluate client's level of orientation and emotional response.

    _____ _____ _____ _____

• Identify unexpected outcomes and intervene as necessary.

    _____ _____ _____ _____

• Record and report intervention and client's response.

    _____ _____ _____ _____

Performance Checklist: Skill 26.4

Using a Rotokinetic Bed

	S	U	NP	Comments

Assessment

1. Identify clients who require complete immobilization and continuous skeletal alignment. ___ ___ ___ _____

2. Carefully inspect the skin for evidence of pressure. ___ ___ ___ _____

3. Assess the client's level of consciousness, orientation, equilibrium, and anxiety. ___ ___ ___ _____

4. Assess client's breath sounds, blood pressure, height, and weight. ___ ___ ___ _____

5. Assess the client's and family members' understanding of and response to the Rotokinetic bed. ___ ___ ___ _____

6. Review medical orders. ___ ___ ___ _____

Implementation

1. Use Standard Protocol. ___ ___ ___ _____

2. Premedicate client 30 minutes before transfer if needed. ___ ___ ___ _____

3. Place Rotokinetic bed in horizontal position and remove all bolsters, straps, and supports. Close posterior hatches. ___ ___ ___ _____

4. Unplug electrical cord. Lock gatch. ___ ___ ___ _____

5. Maintaining proper alignment, transfer client to Rotokinetic bed. ___ ___ ___ _____

6. Secure thoracic panels, bolsters, head and knee packs, and safety straps. ___ ___ ___ _____

7. Cover client with top sheet. ___ ___ ___ _____

8. Plug bed in. ___ ___ ___ _____

9. Have company representative set rotational angle as ordered by the physician. Monitor client's BP. ___ ___ ___ _____

10. Increase degree of rotation gradually according to client's ability to tolerate it. ___ ___ ___ _____

Nurse Alert: The bed must be stopped for CPR and bedside procedures.

11. Provide adequate space for caregivers and family to move around the bed to facilitate communication. Reassure client that he or she will not fall, although he or she may feel lightheaded or as if falling.   ____ ____ ____ _____

12. To stop the bed, permit bed to rotate to the desired position, turn the motor off, and push knob into a lock position. If necessary the bed can be manually repositioned.   ____ ____ ____ _____

Nurse Alert: Keep bed stopped no more than 30 minutes. Manual rotation must be done slowly.

13. Use Completion Protocol.   ____ ____ ____ _____

Evaluation

1. Monitor condition of skin, status of ulcers, and musculoskeletal alignment every 2 hours to determine changes in skin and effectiveness of Rotokinetic therapy.   ____ ____ ____ _____

2. Inspect pressure ulcers for healing.   ____ ____ ____ _____

3. Observe alignment and range of motion.   ____ ____ ____ _____

4. Auscultate lung sounds.   ____ ____ ____ _____

5. Monitor LOC every shift and prn.   ____ ____ ____ _____

6. Ask if client feels nausea or dizziness.   ____ ____ ____ _____

7. Monitor blood pressure.   ____ ____ ____ _____

• Identify unexpected outcomes and intervene as necessary.   ____ ____ ____ _____

• Record and report intervention and client's response.   ____ ____ ____ _____

Performance Checklist: Skill 26.5

Using a Bariatric Bed

	S	U	NP	Comments

Assessment

1. Determine client's need for bed based on height and weight. ____ ____ ____ _____

2. Assess condition of skin. Note condition of skin between skinfolds. Note potential pressure sites. ____ ____ ____ _____

3. Assess client's and family members' understanding of purpose of bed. ____ ____ ____ _____

4. Review client's medical orders. ____ ____ ____ _____

Implementation

1. Use Standard Protocol. ____ ____ ____ _____

2. Position four to six persons around the stretcher or bed to allow a distribution of the client's weight during the lift. ____ ____ ____ _____

Nurse Alert: A mechanical lift may be needed.

3. Place a pull sheet under the client and transfer safely. ____ ____ ____ _____

4. Position the client for comfort with hand controls and trapeze bar within reach. ____ ____ ____ _____

5. Encourage client to initiate frequent position changes and to move about in the bed as much as possible. ____ ____ ____ _____

6. Use Completion Protocol. ____ ____ ____ _____

Evaluation

1. Observe client's ability to manipulate the bed and change position independently. ____ ____ ____ _____

2. Evaluate risk for injury. ____ ____ ____ _____

3. Inspect for skin breakdown q8h. ____ ____ ____ _____

• Identify unexpected outcomes and intervene as necessary. ____ ____ ____ _____

• Record and report intervention and client's response. ____ ____ ____ _____

Performance Checklist: Skill 27.1

Range-of-Motion Exercises

	S	U	NP	Comments

Assessment

1. Review client's chart for physician orders, medical diagnosis, past medical history, and client's progress. _____ _____ _____ _____

2. Obtain data on baseline joint function—ability to perform ROM and limitations. _____ _____ _____ _____

3. Assess client's readiness to learn. Explain all rationales for the ROM exercise and what specific exercises will be performed. _____ _____ _____ _____

4. Assess client's level of comfort (on a scale of 0-10) before exercising. _____ _____ _____ _____

Implementation

1. Use Standard Protocol.

2. Wear gloves (only if there is wound drainage or skin lesions). _____ _____ _____ _____

3. Assist the client to a comfortable position, preferably sitting or lying down. _____ _____ _____ _____

4. Support joint by holding distal and proximal areas adjacent to joint, by cradling distal portion of extremity, or by using cupped hand to support joint. _____ _____ _____ _____

5. Begin following exercises in sequence outlined. Each movement should be repeated five times during exercise period. _____ _____ _____ _____

Nurse Alert: Stop if at any time the client complains of pain, there is resistance, or if there is muscle spasm.

  a. Neck
    (1) *Flexion:* Bring chin to rest on chest. _____ _____ _____ _____
    (2) *Extension:* Return head to erect position. _____ _____ _____ _____
    (3) *Hyperextension:* Bend head as far back as possible. _____ _____ _____ _____
    (4) *Lateral flexion:* Tilt head as far as possible toward each shoulder. _____ _____ _____ _____
    (5) *Rotation:* Rotate head in circular motion (best done in sitting position). _____ _____ _____ _____

(6) Turn head side to side. ___ ___ ___ _____

b. Shoulder

(1) *Flexion:* Raise arm from side position
forward to above head. ___ ___ ___ _____

(2) *Extension:* Return arm to position
at side of body. ___ ___ ___ _____

(3) *Hyperextension:* Move arm behind
body, keeping elbow straight. ___ ___ ___ _____

(4) *Abduction:* Raise arm to side to
position above head with palm
away from head. ___ ___ ___ _____

(5) *Adduction:* Lower arm sideways and
across body as far as possible. ___ ___ ___ _____

(6) *External rotation:* With elbow flexed,
move arm until thumb is upward
and lateral to head. ___ ___ ___ _____

(7) *Internal rotation:* With elbow flexed,
rotate shoulder by moving arm until
thumb is turned inward and toward
back. ___ ___ ___ _____

(8) *Circumduction:* Move arm in a full
circle. ___ ___ ___ _____

c. Elbow

(1) *Flexion:* Bend elbow so that lower
arm moves toward its shoulder joint
and hand is level with shoulder. ___ ___ ___ _____

(2) *Extension:* Straighten elbow by
owering hand. ___ ___ ___ _____

(3) *Hyperextension:* Bend lower arm
back as far as possible. ___ ___ ___ _____

d. Forearm

(1) *Supination:* Turn lower arm and
hand so that palm is up. ___ ___ ___ _____

(2) *Pronation:* Turn lower arm so that
palm is down. ___ ___ ___ _____

e. Wrist

(1) *Flexion:* Move palm toward inner
aspect of forearm. ___ ___ ___ _____

(2) *Extension:* Move palm so fingers,
hands, and forearm are in the same
plane. ___ ___ ___ _____

(3) *Hyperextension:* Bring dorsal surface
of hand back as far as possible. ___ ___ ___ _____

(4) *Abduction (radial flexion):* Bend
wrist medically toward thumb. ___ ___ ___ _____

(5) *Abduction (ulnar flexion):* Bend wrist
laterally toward fifth finger. ___ ___ ___ _____

f. Fingers

(1) *Flexion:* Make fist. ___ ___ ___ _____

(2) *Extension:* Straighten fingers. ___ ___ ___ _____

(3) *Hyperextension:* Bend fingers back as
far as possible. ___ ___ ___ _____

(4) *Abduction:* Spread fingers apart. ___ ___ ___ _____

	S	U	NP	Comments

(5) *Adduction:* Bring fingers together. ____ ____ ____ _____

g. Thumb

   (1) *Flexion:* Move thumb across palmar surface of hand. ____ ____ ____ _____

   (2) *Extension:* Move thumb straight away from hand. ____ ____ ____ _____

   (3) *Abduction:* Extend thumb laterally (usually done when placing fingers in abduction and adduction). ____ ____ ____ _____

   (4) *Adduction:* Move thumb back toward hand. ____ ____ ____ _____

   (5) *Opposition:* Touch thumb to each finger of same hand. ____ ____ ____ _____

h. Hip

   (1) *Flexion:* Move leg forward and up. ____ ____ ____ _____

   (2) *Extension:* Move leg back beside other leg. ____ ____ ____ _____

   (3) *Hyperextension:* Move leg behind body (best done standing or lying on abdomen). ____ ____ ____ _____

   (4) *Abduction:* Move leg laterally away from body. ____ ____ ____ _____

   (5) *Adduction:* Move leg back toward medial position and beyond if possible. ____ ____ ____ _____

   (6) *Internal rotation:* Turn foot and leg toward other leg. ____ ____ ____ _____

   (7) *External rotation:* Turn foot and leg away from other leg. ____ ____ ____ _____

   (8) *Circumduction:* Move leg in circle. ____ ____ ____ _____

i. Knee

   (1) *Flexion:* Bring heel toward back of thigh (done with hip flexion). ____ ____ ____ _____

   (2) *Extension:* Return leg to straight position on bed. ____ ____ ____ _____

j. Ankle

   (1) *Plantar flexion:* Move foot so toes are pointed downward. ____ ____ ____ _____

   (2) *Dorsal flexion:* Move foot so toes are pointed upward. ____ ____ ____ _____

k. Foot

   (1) *Inversion:* Turn sole of foot medially. ____ ____ ____ _____

   (2) *Eversion:* Turn sole of foot laterally. ____ ____ ____ _____

   (3) *Flexion:* Curl toes downward. ____ ____ ____ _____

   (4) *Extension:* Straighten toes. ____ ____ ____ _____

   (5) *Abduction:* Spread toes apart. ____ ____ ____ _____

   (6) *Adduction:* Bring toes together. ____ ____ ____ _____

6. Use Completion Protocol. ____ ____ ____ _____

Evaluation

1. Observe client performing ROM activities. ____ ____ ____ _____

2. Measure ROM in degrees (e.g., 45°) and compare to normal ROM for that joint. ____ ____ ____ _____

	S	U	NP	Comments

3. Ask client to rate discomfort using pain scale.

4. Evaluate client/caregiver ability to perform ROM.

- Identify unexpected outcomes and intervene as necessary.

- Report and record intervention and client's response.

Performance Checklist: Skill 27.2

Continuous Passive Motion Machine (for Client with Total Knee Replacement)

	S	U	NP	Comments

Assessment

1. Check the machine for electrical safety. ____ ____ ____ _____

2. Assess the setup of the machine before placing on bed: check the stability of the frame, the flexion/extension controls, speed controls, and the on/off switch. ____ ____ ____ _____

3. Assess the client for comfort before and during use. ____ ____ ____ _____

4. Assess client's baseline HR and BP. ____ ____ ____ _____

5. Assess the client's ability and willingness to learn about the CPM machine. ____ ____ ____ _____

6. Assess client's ROM before therapy begins. ____ ____ ____ _____

Implementation

1. Use Standard Protocol. ____ ____ ____ _____

2. Provide analgesia 20-30 miutes before CPM. ____ ____ ____ _____

3. Wear gloves (if wound drainage is present). ____ ____ ____ _____

4. Test all CPM controls to make sure they are functional. ____ ____ ____ _____

5. Demonstrate machine to client. ____ ____ ____ _____

6. Stop the machine in full extension. ____ ____ ____ _____

7. Place client's leg in the machine, being sure to support above, below, and at knee. ____ ____ ____ _____

8. Fit CPM machine to client by lengthening and shortening appropriate section of the CPM frame. ____ ____ ____ _____

9. Align client's knee joint (bend of the knee) with the machine knee hinge, then position the client's knee 2 cm below knee joint line of the CPM. ____ ____ ____ _____

10. Center client's leg in the machine. ____ ____ ____ _____

11. Adjust the foot support to approximately 20 degrees of dorsiflexion to prevent footdrop. ____ ____ ____ _____

	S	U	NP	Comments

12. When client's leg is in correct position, secure the Velcro straps across lower extremity (thigh) and top of foot.

13. Start CPM machine. Watch at least two full cycles of prescribed flexion and extension. Remove and discard gloves, if worn, and wash hands.

14. Make sure client is comfortable. Provide client with the on/off switch. Instruct to use only if CPM seems to be malfunctioning.

15. Use Completion Protocol.

16. Periodically reassess client's comfort level and proper function of machine.

Evaluation

1. Ask client to keep a log of when the CPM machine is in use, with times and dates.

2. Observe client at the initial onset of an increase in the flexion of the machine.

3. Ask client to rate comfort level.

4. Measure joint ROM achieved with CPM machine.

5. Observe skin every 2 hours for signs of breakdown.

• Identify unexpected outcomes and intervene as necessary.

• Report and record intervention and client's response.

Name _____ Date _____ Instructor's Name _____

Performance Checklist: Skill 28.1

Care of the Client in Skin Traction

	S	U	NP	Comments

Assessment

1. Assess client's knowledge of the reason for traction.

2. Assess integrity and condition of skin to be placed in traction.

3. Assess client's overall health condition, including degree of mobility, ability to perform activities of daily living (ADLs), and current medical conditions.

4. Assess client's position in bed: supine, perpendicular to the ends of the bed, with the affected limb in proper body alignment.

5. Assess client's level of pain and need for analgesics before procedure begins.

6. Assess neurovascular status of the extremity.

Implementation

1. Use Standard Protocol.

2. Position client supine and nearly flat with no more than 30 degrees of elevation, with the affected leg halfway between the edge of the bed and middle of the bed.

3. Wash affected leg (or legs) gently and pat dry.

Nurse Alert: Do not apply over damaged skin. Ensure that skin traction is not too tight or too loose.

4. Apply foam boot, moleskin, or elastic bandages to affected leg, proceeding distal to proximal.

5. Attach weight to boot gradually and gently at the end of the bed.

Nurse Alert: Avoid pressure to peroneal nerve at neck of fibula when applying Buck's traction.

6. Inspect traction setup. Ropes are tied securely in knots, passed through grooves of pulleys to weights, are not frayed, and are hanging freely.

	S	U	NP	Comments

7. Assess neurovascular status of extremity distal to the traction, including skin color and temperature, capillary refill, presence of distal pulses, sensation, and client's ability to move digits, every 30 minutes times two and every 4 hours while traction is in place.

Nurse Alert: Compare with uninvolved extremity to determine if deficit is related to traction wrap.

8. Release traction boot every 4 to 8 hours and provide skin care according to physician's orders.

9. Use Completion Protocol.

Evaluation

1. Evaluate traction setup.

2. Monitor condition of skin for pressure, color changes, edema, or tenderness.

3. Evaluate client's ability to perform ADLs.

4. Ask client to rate comfort level.

5. Evaluate neurovascular status.

6. Observe client's use of trapeze and overhead frame with unaffected limbs to reposition self correctly.

• Identify unexpected outcomes and intervene as necessary.

• Record and report intervention and client's response.

Name _____ Date _____ Instructor's Name _____

Performance Checklist: Skill 28.2

Care of the Client in Skeletal Traction and Pin Site Care

	S	U	NP	Comments

Assessment

1. Assess client's knowledge of the reason for traction, including nonverbal behavior and responses. ____ ____ ____ _____

2. Assess integrity and condition of skin over bony prominences and under devices in use. ____ ____ ____ _____

3. Assess client's overall health condition, including degree of mobility, ability to perform ADLs, and current medical conditions. ____ ____ ____ _____

4. Assess client's level of pain and need for analgesics before procedure begins. ____ ____ ____ _____

5. Assess traction setup. ____ ____ ____ _____

6. Assess neurovascular status of extremity. ____ ____ ____ _____

7. Assess client's mobility. ____ ____ ____ _____

8. Assess pin sites for signs of infection. ____ ____ ____ _____

9. Assess for respiratory dysfunction. ____ ____ ____ _____

Implementation

1. Use Standard Protocol. ____ ____ ____ _____

2. Inspect traction setup. Check the four P's of traction maintenance.

Nurse Alert: Irreversible tissue death occurs within 4-12 hours.

3. Monitor neurovascular status of distal aspects of involved extremities in comparison with corresponding body part every 2 hours for the first 24 hours and every 4 to 12 hours thereafter (according to agency policy). ____ ____ ____ _____

4. Provide pin site care according to hospital policy or physician's orders. ____ ____ ____ _____
   a. Apply gloves. Remove gauze dressings from around pins and discard in receptacle. ____ ____ ____ _____
   b. Inspect sites for drainage or inflammation. ____ ____ ____ _____

	S	U	NP	Comments

c. Prepare supplies and apply new gloves.

d. Clean each pin site with prescribed solution by placing sterile applicator close to the pin and cleaning away from the insertion site. Dispose of applicator.

e. Repeat process for each pin site.

f. Using a sterile applicator, apply a small amount of topical antibiotic ointment (check for physician's orders or hospital policy).

g. Cover with a sterile 2 × 2 split gauze dressing or leave site open to air (OTA) as prescribed or according to hospital policy. Remove and discard gloves and wash hands.

5. Inspect skin over bony prominences for signs of pressure and lightly massage q2h unless skin breakdown is evident.

6. Assess risk for pressure ulcers.

7. Monitor respiratory status every shift.

8. Assess level of discomfort and provide nonpharmacological and pharmacological relief as indicated.

Nurse Alert: Never ignore a client's complaint.

9. Encourage active and passive exercises and use of unaffected extremities for ADLs. Encourage use of trapeze bar for repositioning in bed.

10. Provide a fracture pan for elimination.

11. Use Completion Protocol.

Evaluation

1. Determine client's response to traction and immobilization.

2. Monitor skin condition.

3. Observe client's participation in ADLs.

4. Ask client to rate comfort level.

5. Monitor neurovascular status of extremities.

6. Evaluate for systemic infection or local inflammation at pin sites.

• Identify unexpected outcomes and intervene as necessary.

• Record and report intervention and client's response.

Performance Checklist: Skill 28.3

Care of the Client During Cast Application

	S	U	NP	Comments

Assessment

1. Assess client's health status, focusing on factors that may affect wound healing. ____ ____ ____ _____

2. Assess client's ability to cooperate and level of understanding concerning the casting procedure. ____ ____ ____ _____

3. Assess condition of the skin that will be under the cast. ____ ____ ____ _____

4. Assess neurovascular status of the area to be casted, including motor/sensory function, skin color and temperature, and capillary refill. ____ ____ ____ _____

5. Assess client's pain status using a scale of 0 to 10. ____ ____ ____ _____

6. Consult with physician to determine the extent to which client will be able to use the casted body part. ____ ____ ____ _____

Implementation

1. Use Standard Protocol. ____ ____ ____ _____

2. Administer analgesic before cast application: orally (PO) 30 to 40 minutes prior; intramuscularly (IM) 20 to 30 minutes prior; intravenously (IV) 2 to 5 minutes prior. ____ ____ ____ _____

3. Apply gloves. Position client and injured extremity as desired, depending on type of cast to be used and area to be casted. ____ ____ ____ _____

4. Prepare skin that will be enclosed in the cast. Change any dressing (if present), and cleanse the skin with mild soap and water. ____ ____ ____ _____

Nurse Alert: Clients with skin damage or lesions may not be candidates for casting.

5. Assist with application of padding material around body part to be casted. Avoid wrinkles or uneven thicknesses. ____ ____ ____ _____

	S	U	NP	Comments

6. Hold body part or parts to be casted or assist with preparation of casting materials.
   a. Plaster cast: Mark the end of the roll by folding one corner of the material under itself. Hold plaster roll under water in a plastic-lined bucket or basin until bubbles stop, then squeeze slightly and hand roll to person applying the cast.
   b. Synthetic cast: Submerge cast roll in lukewarm water for 10 to 15 seconds. Squeeze to remove excess water.

7. Continue to hold the body parts as necessary as the cast is applied or supply additional rolls of casting tape as needed.

8. Provide walking heel, brace, bar, or other material to stabilize the cast as requested by the physician.

Nurse Alert: Do not use abduction bar as a handle for positioning the client.

9. Assist with "finishing" the cast by folding the edge of the stockinette down over the cast to provide a smooth edge. A dampened plaster roll is unrolled over the stockinette to hold it in place.

10. Using scissors, trim the cast around fingers, toes, or the thumb as necessary. Remove and discard gloves and wash hands.

11. Elevate the casted tissues on cloth-covered pillows or placed in a sling. Avoid complete encasing of the cast. Allow to air dry.

12. Inform client to notify caregiver of alteration in sensation or movement.

13. Assist client with transfer to stretcher or wheelchair for return to unit, or prepare for discharge, using palms of hands to support casted area.

Nurse Alert: Client with large-limb or wet spica cast requires three people to assist in turning and transfer.

14. Review all home care instructions with client/caregiver(s).

15. Clean used equipment and return to usual storage area.

16. Explain need to keep cast exposed until drying is complete.

	S	U	NP	Comments

17. Have client turn every 2 or 3 hours when a body jacket or a hip spica cast is applied. _____ _____ _____ _____

18. Use Completion Protocol. _____ _____ _____ _____

Evaluation

1. Evaluate skin condition and neurovascular status of casted area. _____ _____ _____ _____

2. Palpate temperature of tissues around casted area. _____ _____ _____ _____

3. Palpate pulses distal to cast. _____ _____ _____ _____

4. Inspect condition of cast. _____ _____ _____ _____

5. Observe for edema distal to cast. _____ _____ _____ _____

6. Monitor client for signs of pain or anxiety. _____ _____ _____ _____

7. Observe client performing ADLs and ROM. _____ _____ _____ _____

8. Ask client to describe cast care. _____ _____ _____ _____

9. Determine client's/caregiver's ability to perform cast care. _____ _____ _____ _____

• Identify unexpected outcomes and intervene as necessary. _____ _____ _____ _____

• Record and report intervention and client's response. _____ _____ _____ _____

Performance Checklist: Skill 28.4

Care of the Client During Cast Removal

	S	U	NP	Comments

Assessment

1. Assess client's understanding and ability to cooperate with cast removal. ____ ____ ____ _____

2. Assess client's readiness for cast removal. ____ ____ ____ _____

3. Ask if client feels itching or irritation under the cast. ____ ____ ____ _____

Implementation

1. Use Standard Protocol. ____ ____ ____ _____

2. Assist with positioning of client to prevent skin injury. ____ ____ ____ _____

3. Apply gloves. Describe the physical sensations to expect during cast removal. ____ ____ ____ _____

4. Describe the expected appearance of the extremity (scaly dead cells). ____ ____ ____ _____

5. Explain the loud noise of the cast saw. ____ ____ ____ _____

6. Stay with client, and explain progress of procedure as cast is removed. ____ ____ ____ _____

7. Inspect tissues underlying the cast after removal. ____ ____ ____ _____

8. If skin is intact, apply cold water enzyme wash (if available) to skin and leave on for 15 to 20 minutes. Mild soap and water may also be used. Do not scrub the skin. ____ ____ ____ _____

9. Gently wash off enzyme wash. Immerse tissues in basin or tub, if possible, to assist in dead cell removal. ____ ____ ____ _____

10. Pat extremity dry and apply thin coat of skin lotion. ____ ____ ____ _____

11. Explain and write out skin care procedures after cast removal to client. ____ ____ ____ _____

12. Obtain physician's order to perform active and passive ROM, and clarify level of activity allowed. ____ ____ ____ _____

	S	U	NP	Comments

13. Assist in transfer of client for return to unit or discharge. ___ ___ ___ _____

14. Clean all equipment. Dispose of cast and materials according to universal precautions. ___ ___ ___ _____

15. Use Completion Protocol. ___ ___ ___ _____

Evaluation

1. Ask client to demonstrate ability to perform ADLs and skin care. ___ ___ ___ _____

2. Inspect skin for pressure areas, erythema, or trauma. ___ ___ ___ _____

3. Observe client perform skin care. ___ ___ ___ _____

• Identify unexpected outcomes and intervene as necessary. ___ ___ ___ _____

• Record and report intervention and client's response. ___ ___ ___ _____

Performance Checklist: Skill 28.5

Care of the Client with an Immobilization Device (Brace, Splint, Sling)

	S	U	NP	Comments

Assessment

1. Review client's chart, including medical history, previous and current activity level, and description of the condition requiring bracing or splinting. ____ ____ ____ _____

2. Assess client's previous experience with braces or splints. ____ ____ ____ _____

3. Assess client's understanding of reason for brace/splint, care of, application of, and schedule of wear. ____ ____ ____ _____

4. Assess client's risk for skin breakdown because of bracing/splinting or immobilization. ____ ____ ____ _____

5. Assess client's level of pain.

6. Refer to occupational or physical therapy consult to determine type of brace to be used, desired position, and amount of activity and movement permitted. ____ ____ ____ _____

7. Assess client's additional need for an assistive device such as a cane, walker, or crutches. ____ ____ ____ _____

Implementation

1. Use Standard Protocol. ____ ____ ____ _____

2. Explain reasons for the brace or splint, and demonstrate how the device works. ____ ____ ____ _____

3. Assist the client to a comfortable position, preferably sitting or lying down. ____ ____ ____ _____

4. Prepare the skin that will be enclosed in the brace/splint by cleaning the skin with soap and water; rinse, pat dry, and change any dressings (if present). If applying a back brace, put a thin cotton shirt or gown on the client. ____ ____ ____ _____

5. Inspect the device for wear, damage, or rough edges. ____ ____ ____ _____

	S	U	NP	Comments

6. Apply the brace/splint as directed by physician, orthotist, physical therapist, or occupational therapist.

7. Teach the client the prescribed schedule of wear and allowed activities while in the brace/splint as directed by physician, physical therapist, or occupational therapist.

8. Reinforce the signs of skin breakdown, pressure, or rubbing to report.

9. Teach the client how to care for the brace/splint (storage and cleaning).

10. Assist client to ambulate with brace/splint in place.

11. Have the client apply and remove the brace/splint.

12. Use Completion Protocol.

Evaluation

1. Inspect areas of skin underneath the brace/splint.

2. Observe client's use of brace/splint.

3. Ask client to rate comfort level.

4. Palpate pulse and test sensation distal to brace/splint.

5. Observe client perform ADLs while wearing brace/splint.

- Identify unexpected outcomes and intervene as necessary.

- Record and report intervention and client's response.

Performance Checklist: Procedural Guideline 28-1

Sling Application

	S	U	NP	Comments
1. Use Standard Protocol.	____	____	____	_____
2. Follow directions on package for application of a commercial sling.	____	____	____	_____
3. For triangular bandage, position one end of the bandage over the shoulder of the unaffected arm.	____	____	____	_____
4. Take the remaining bandage and place the material against the chest, then under and over the affected arm, cradling the arm.	____	____	____	_____
5. Position the pointed end of the triangle toward the elbow.	____	____	____	_____
6. Tie the two ends of the triangle at the side of the neck.	____	____	____	_____
7. Fold the pointed end of the sling at the elbow in the front and secure with a safety pin, closing the end of the sling.	____	____	____	_____
8. Adjust the length of the sling by adjusting the amount of material in the knot.	____	____	____	_____
9. Ensure the sling supports the limb comfortably without interfering with circulation.	____	____	____	_____
10. Assess neurovascular status after 20 to 30 minutes. Continue to monitor every 4 hours. Readjust sling as necessary.	____	____	____	_____
11. Use Completion Protocol.	____	____	____	_____

Name _____ Date _____ Instructor's Name _____

Performance Checklist: Skill 29.5

Transfusions with Blood Products

| | S | U | NP | Comments |

Assessment

1. Verify physician's order for type of blood product, length of transfusion (up to 4 hours for whole blood or red blood cells), and medications to be given. _____ _____ _____ _____

2. Assess client's transfusion history, including previous transfusion reaction. Verify that type and crossmatch has been completed within 72 hours of transfusion and, if applicable, that consent for transfusion is signed. _____ _____ _____ _____

3. Establish that client has a patent large-bore IV catheter with positive blood return. _____ _____ _____ _____

4. Assess pretransfusion, baseline vital signs. If client is febrile, notify physician before initiating transfusion (check agency policy). _____ _____ _____ _____

5. Assess client's medication schedule. _____ _____ _____ _____

Implementation

1. Use Standard Protocol. _____ _____ _____ _____

2. Obtain blood bag from laboratory following agency protocol. Blood transfusions must be initiated 15 to 30 minutes after release from laboratory. _____ _____ _____ _____

3. Open blood administration set and prime the tubing with normal saline, completely filling filter with saline. Maintain sterility of system and close lower clamp. _____ _____ _____ _____

Nurse Alert: IV medications cannot be added to blood bag or infused through transfusion administration set.

4. Have client void or empty urinary drainage collection container. _____ _____ _____ _____

5. With another registered nurse or licensed nurse, correctly verify blood product and identify client (check agency policy). _____ _____ _____ _____

335

a. Client's name, identification number, and birth date

____ ____ ____ _____

b. Client's name, identification number, and birth date with forms from blood bank and with physician's order in client's record

____ ____ ____ _____

c. Client's blood group and Rh type

____ ____ ____ _____

d. Crossmatch compatibility

____ ____ ____ _____

e. Donor's blood group and Rh type

____ ____ ____ _____

f. Unit and hospital number

____ ____ ____ _____

g. Expiration date and time on blood unit

____ ____ ____ _____

h. Type of blood component is correct component ordered by physician.

____ ____ ____ _____

Nurse Alert: Most serious transfusion reactions occur from identification errors and can be life threatening.

6. Apply gloves. Inspect blood product for signs of leakage or unusual appearance, including clots, bubbles, or purplish color. Gently invert bag 2 or 3 times.

____ ____ ____ _____

7. Attach blood product by inserting spike of Y tubing located next to normal saline. Close normal saline clamp above filter and open clamp above filter to blood product.

____ ____ ____ _____

8. Review with client the purpose of transfusion. Ask client to report immediately any signs and symptoms (during or after transfusion), including chills, low back pain, shortness of breath, nausea, excessive perspiration, rash, or even a vague sense of uneasiness.

____ ____ ____ _____

Nurse Alert: A transfusion reaction is an emergency.

9. Connect normal saline–primed blood administration set directly to client's IV site. Remove and discard gloves and wash hands.

____ ____ ____ _____

10. Open lower clamp and regulate blood infusion to allow only 10 to 24 ml to infuse in the first 15 minutes. Remain with client.

____ ____ ____ _____

11. Obtain vital signs 15 minutes after initiation of transfusion.

____ ____ ____ _____

12. Reregulate flow clamp if there is no transfusion reaction, and infuse the remaining volume of blood as ordered by physician. Packed red blood cells are usually infused over 2 hours and whole

	S	U	NP	Comments

blood over 3 to 4 hours. Check blood
tubing package for correct drop factor.

   ___ ___ ___   _____

**Nurse Alert: Blood must be infused within 4 hours
or discarded to minimize risk of bacterial infection.**

13. Continue to monitor vital signs per agency
policy and procedure during transfusion.

   ___ ___ ___   _____

14. After blood has infused, close roller clamp
above filter to blood and open normal saline.

   ___ ___ ___   _____

15. Infuse normal saline until tubing is
completely clear.

   ___ ___ ___   _____

16. Apply gloves. Discontinue transfusion and
blood administration set.

   ___ ___ ___   _____

17. Follow standard precautions and agency
protocol for disposal of old blood bags and
tubing. Remove and discard gloves and
wash hands.

   ___ ___ ___   _____

18. Apply injection cap and flush existing
IV line, or restart IV fluids as ordered only
after assessing IV site for patency and signs
and symptoms of phlebitis. If transfusing
more than one unit of blood or blood
product, maintain normal saline via blood
administration set at KVO rate until
second unit is started. Change
administration set after each unit or after
4 hours.

   ___ ___ ___   _____

19. Use Completion Protocol.

   ___ ___ ___   _____

Evaluation

1. Observe for transfusion reaction: chills,
fever, itching, hives, dyspnea, tachycardia,
hypotension.

   ___ ___ ___   _____

2. Monitor I&O, laboratory values, and
client response.

   ___ ___ ___   _____

3. Observe for signs of physical or emotional
stress during transfusion.

   ___ ___ ___   _____

4. Monitor IV site and status of infusion
every time vital signs are taken.

   ___ ___ ___   _____

5. Ask client to describe purpose, benefit,
and risk of transfusion.

   ___ ___ ___   _____

• Identify unexpected outcomes and
intervene as necessary.

   ___ ___ ___   _____

• Record and report intervention and
client's response.

   ___ ___ ___   _____

Performance Checklist: Skill 30.1

Monitoring Fluid Balance

	S	U	NP	Comments

Assessment

1. Consult the medical record or complete a nursing history with the client and family to identify risk factors for fluid volume imbalances.

2. Monitor cardiovascular status for changes.

3. Check daily weights and I&O.

4. Inspect oral mucous membranes.

5. Inspect skin for temperature and moisture.

6. Assess mental status and level of consciousness.

7. Monitor laboratory values.

8. Assess client's and family's understanding of fluid imbalances and the importance of accurate assessment data.

Implementation

1. Use Standard Protocol.

2. Provide oral hygiene every 2 to 4 hours and keep lips moist with petrolatum jelly.

3. Monitor daily weights for trends toward normal.

4. Provide careful skin care.

5. Provide client safety and position changes.

6. Implement specific interventions to improve fluid status
   a. Fluid volume deficit (FVD)
      (1) Encourage fluids if oral intake is not restricted.
      (2) Monitor IV therapy carefully for overload including daily weights, I&O, and cardiopulmonary status.

Nurse Alert: Assess the client frequently for FVE if rapid rates of IV infusion are required, especially in the presence of cardiac, renal, or neurological problems.

	S	U	NP	Comments

b. Fluid volume excess (FVE)
   (1) Monitor IV therapy for appropriate rate of administration and effectiveness. _____ _____ _____ _____
   (2) Elevate the head of the bed and provide oxygen as indicated. _____ _____ _____ _____
   (3) Administer medications, such as diuretics, as prescribed. _____ _____ _____ _____
   (4) Restrict fluids to 1200 to 1500 ml/day. _____ _____ _____ _____

7. Monitor output for trends toward normal fluid balance. _____ _____ _____ _____

8. Monitor appropriate laboratory values. _____ _____ _____ _____

9. Use Completion Protocol. _____ _____ _____ _____

Evaluation

1. Conduct ongoing assessment to determine whether fluid imbalance has been corrected. _____ _____ _____ _____

2. Evaluate effectiveness of corrective actions. _____ _____ _____ _____

3. Evaluate for possible complications of overcorrection. _____ _____ _____ _____

- Identify unexpected outcomes and intervene as necessary. _____ _____ _____ _____

- Record and report intervention and client's response. _____ _____ _____ _____

Performance Checklist: Skill 30.2

Monitoring Electrolyte Balance

	S	U	NP	Comments

Assessment

1. Consult the medical record, or complete a nursing history with the client and family to identify risk factors for electrolyte imbalances.

2. Consider current illness or disease processes, health practices, and dietary restrictions.

3. Check laboratory results to identify abnormal electrolyte levels.

4. Assess client's and family's understanding of the risk for electrolyte imbalances.

Implementation

1. Use Standard Protocol.

2. Assess for sodium imbalance: Identify conditions that contribute to sodium imbalance.
   a. *Hyponatremia:* Assess for evidence of hyponatremia (serum sodium level less than 135 mEq/L).
      (1) Assess for abdominal cramps, nausea, and vomiting.
      (2) Assess mental status for personality change, irritability, apprehension, anxiety, convulsions, or coma.
      (3) Monitor vital signs for weak, rapid pulse and hypotension.
   b. *Hypernatremia:* Assess for evidence of hyponatremia (sodium level greater than 145 mEq/L).
      (1) Assess for thirst, lethargy, weakness, and irritability.
      (2) Inspect mouth for dry tongue and mucous membranes.
      (3) Assess for dry, flushed skin and thirst.
      (4) Monitor urine output for oliguria or anuria.
   c. Provide comfort and safety measures, including preparation for potential convulsions in severe cases.

    d. Refer to dietitian if a low-sodium diet is prescribed; teach the client ways to consume less salt and sodium.

        (1) Read the nutrition labels and minimize the use of processed foods. Look for foods with reduced or no sodium.

        (2) Use fresh and plain frozen vegetables.

        (3) Request no added salt when eating out or traveling.

        (4) Use spices and herbs rather than salt to enhance flavor.

        (5) Avoid condiments such as pickles, olives, soy sauces, and other items high in sodium.

        (6) Choose fresh fruits and vegetables as snacks rather than salted chips, nuts, or popcorn.

        (7) Avoid over-the-counter medications that contain sodium.

3. Assess for potassium imbalance: Identify conditions that contribute to potassium imbalance.

    a. *Hypokalemia:* Assess for evidence of hypokalemia (serum potassium level less than 3.5 mEq/L).

        (1) Assess vital signs for a weak, irregular pulse; shallow respirations; and hypotension.

        (2) Assess electrocardiogram (ECG) changes.

Nurse Alert: Severe hypokalemia can result in death from cardiac or respiratory arrest.

        (3) Assess for generalized weakness, decreased muscle tone, decreased reflexes, or fatigue.

        (4) Assess abdomen for decreased bowel sounds and abdominal distention.

        (5) Assess extremities for muscle cramps and paresthesias.

    b. Maintain adequate dietary intake of potassium.

    c. Administer IV fluids with as ordered.

Nurse Alert: The rate of IV fluids with KCl should not exceed 20 mEq of potassium/hour.

    d. *Hyperkalemia:* Assess for evidence of hyperkalemia (serum potassium greater than 5.5 mEq/L).

        (1) Assess ECG changes.

        (2) Assess for nausea, vomiting, diarrhea, and cramping pain.

(3) Assess for muscle twitching, paresthesias or paralysis, or seizures. ____ ____ ____ _____

e. In the presence of hyperkalemia, collaborate with the physician to prescribe Kayexalate and/or promote the excretion of potassium with dialysis. ____ ____ ____ _____

4. Assess for calcium imbalance: Identify conditions that contribute to calcium imbalance. ____ ____ ____ _____

a. *Hypocalcemia:* Monitor laboratory reports for hypocalcemia (total serum calcium less than 8.5 mg/dl). ____ ____ ____ _____

(1) Assess for muscle cramps, numbness, and tingling in extremities. ____ ____ ____ _____

(2) Assess for ECG changes, laryngeal spasm, or respiratory arrest. ____ ____ ____ _____

(3) Observe for laryngeal spasm and prepare for possible respiratory arrest. ____ ____ ____ _____

Nurse Alert: Severe hypocalcemia is a medical emergency treated with calcium gluconate.

(4) Assess for colicky discomfort or diarrhea. ____ ____ ____ _____

(5) Assess for Chvostek's sign, a contraction of facial muscles in response to a light tap over the facial nerve in front of the ear. ____ ____ ____ _____

(6) Assess for Trousseau's sign, carpal spasm induced by inflating a blood pressure cuff above the systolic pressure for as long as 3 minutes. ____ ____ ____ _____

(7) Prepare for possible seizures and tetany. ____ ____ ____ _____

b. *Hypercalcemia:* Assess laboratory reports for hypercalcemia (total serum calcium greater than 11 mg/dl).

(1) Assess for decreased gastrointestinal motility, including anorexia, nausea, or constipation. ____ ____ ____ _____

(2) Assess for lethargy, muscle weakness, fatigue, and malaise. ____ ____ ____ _____

(3) Assess for confusion, impaired memory, sudden psychosis, or coma. ____ ____ ____ _____

(4) Monitor for weight loss, dehydration, and increased thirst. ____ ____ ____ _____

(5) Assess for hypertension or ECG changes. ____ ____ ____ _____

(6) Assess for decreased muscle strength, hypoventilation, and depressed reflexes. ____ ____ ____ _____

(7) Assess abdomen for hypoactive bowel sounds or paralytic ileus. ____ ____ ____ _____

c. Promote excretion of calcium by increasing fluid intake to 3000 to

343

	S	U	NP	Comments

4000 ml of fluid daily or administration of a loop diuretic as ordered. ___ ___ ___ _____

5. Assess for magnesium imbalance: Identify factors that contribute to magnesium imbalance.

   a. *Hypomagnesemia:* Assess for evidence of magnesium deficit (less than 1.5 mEq/L).

     (1) Assess for hyperactive deep tendon reflexes (DTRs), tremors, and convulsions. ___ ___ ___ _____

     (2) Assess mental status for sudden changes, including confusion. ___ ___ ___ _____

     (3) Monitor for cardiac dysrhythmias. ___ ___ ___ _____

   b. *Hypermagnesemia:* Assess for evidence of magnesium excess (greater than 2.5 mEq/L).

     (1) Assess for hypotension, lethargy, and drowsiness. ___ ___ ___ _____

     (2) Assess for hyporeflexia. ___ ___ ___ _____

     (3) Assess for nausea and vomiting. ___ ___ ___ _____

     (4) Assess for ECG changes. ___ ___ ___ _____

6. Use Completion Protocol. ___ ___ ___ _____

Evaluation

1. Check laboratory values and physical signs to identify trends. ___ ___ ___ _____

2. Monitor for evidence of complications related to treatment. ___ ___ ___ _____

• Identify unexpected outcomes and intervene as necessary. ___ ___ ___ _____

• Record and report intervention and client's response. ___ ___ ___ _____

Performance Checklist: Skill 30.3

Monitoring Acid-Base Balance

	S	U	NP	Comments

Assessment

1. Assess client's risk factors for acid-base imbalances.

2. Assess factors that influence arterial blood gas (ABG) measurements.

3. Identify medications that may affect acid-base balance.

Implementation

1. Use Standard Protocol.

2. Collect ABG sample by arterial puncture.
   a. Select an appropriate site—radial, femoral, or brachial artery commonly used.
   b. Assess collateral blood flow to the hand using Allen's test.
      (1) Have client make a tight fist and raise hand above heart.
      (2) Apply direct pressure to both radial and ulnar arteries.
      (3) Have client lower hand and open hand.
      (4) Release pressure over ulnar artery; observe color of fingers, thumbs, and hand.
   c. Apply gloves. Palpate selected site with fingertips.
   d. Stabilize artery by hyperextending wrist slightly.
   e. Clean area of maximal impulse with alcohol swab, wiping in a circular motion.
   f. Hold needle bevel up and insert at 45-degree angle, observing for blood return.
   g. Stop advancing needle when blood is observed and allow arterial pulsations to pump 2 to 3 ml of blood into the heparinized syringe.
   h. When sampling is complete, hold 2 × 2 gauze pad over puncture site and quickly withdraw needle, applying pressure over and just proximal to puncture site.

S   U   NP   Comments

i. Maintain continuous pressure on and proximal to the site for 3 to 5 minutes longer.

_____ _____ _____ _____

j. Inspect site for signs of bleeding or hematoma formation.

_____ _____ _____ _____

k. Palpate artery distal to puncture site.

_____ _____ _____ _____

l. Expel air bubbles from syringe.

_____ _____ _____ _____

m. Place identification label on syringes, place syringe in ice, and attach appropriate laboratory requisition. Note if the client is receiving supplemental oxygen, and identify the client's temperature.

_____ _____ _____ _____

n. Transport specimen to the laboratory immediately.

_____ _____ _____ _____

3. Interpret ABG report. Check the PaO_2 (norm is 80-100 mm Hg) and the SaO_2 (norm is 95%-100%).

_____ _____ _____ _____

4. Check the pH to determine whether it is alkalotic (greater than 7.45) or acidotic (less than 7.35).

_____ _____ _____ _____

5. Determine the primary cause of the change in the pH. Check the $PaCO_2$ to determine whether it is high, within normal limits, or low (normal is 35-45 mm Hg).

a. If the $PaCO_2$ is high (*respiratory acidosis*), collaborate with other health team members to determine ways to improve the client's ventilation to eliminate excess CO_2.

_____ _____ _____ _____

b. If the $PaCO_2$ is low (*respiratory alkalosis*), collaborate with other health team members to determine ways to promote retention of CO_2.

_____ _____ _____ _____

c. If $PaCO_2$ is normal, the client is ventilating adequately.

_____ _____ _____ _____

6. Check the HCO_3 to determine whether it is high, within normal limits, or low (normal is 22-26 mEq/L).

_____ _____ _____ _____

a. If the HCO_3 is high (*metabolic loss* of acids), collaborate with other health team members to determine ways to minimize the metabolic loss of acids.

_____ _____ _____ _____

b. If the HCO_3 is low and the CO_2 is normal (accumulation of acids caused by a metabolic process), collaborate with health team members to treat the condition.

_____ _____ _____ _____

7. Determine whether there is evidence of the body attempting to compensate for the pH change.

_____ _____ _____ _____

	S	U	NP	Comments

a. If the primary problem is respiratory acidosis (pH less than 7.4 with an elevated pCO_2), the kidneys may compensate by retaining bicarbonate.

b. If the primary problem is metabolic acidosis (pH less than 7.4 with a bicarbonate deficit), the body may compensate by hyperventilating immediately.

c. If the primary problem is respiratory alkalosis (pH greater than 7.4 with low CO_2), the body may compensate by decreasing renal absorption of bicarbonate.

d. If the primary problem is metabolic alkalosis (pH greater than 7.4 with bicarbonate excess), the body may compensate immediately with hypoventilation.

8. Use Completion Protocol.

Evaluation

1. Observe puncture site for bleeding and verify circulation to extremity.

2. Analyze the ABG to determine whether acid-base imbalance has been corrected.

3. Assess for evidence of complications.

- Identify unexpected outcomes and intervene as necessary.

- Record and report intervention and client's response.

Performance Checklist: Skill 31.2

Airway Management: Noninvasive Interventions

	S	U	NP	Comments

Assessment

1. Assess increased work of breathing or inability to clear copious or tenacious secretions by coughing.

2. Assess for shortness of breath, wheezing, use of accessory muscles of respiration, pallor or cyanosis, nasal flaring, snoring respirations, or sleep apnea.

3. Assess client's Sp O_2 with oximetry.

4. Assess for possible sleep apnea.

5. Monitor PEFR initially and with changes in therapy. Assess client's baseline knowledge of PEFR.

Implementation

1. Use Standard Protocol.

2. Correct positioning of client
   a. Sitting: Semi-Fowler's or high Fowler's, sitting on side of bed, or in chair with elbows resting on knees. Clients with COPD may benefit from leaning over table with arms propped up.
   b. Standing: Support client when ambulating, encourage a position that supports client.
   c. Supine: Determine whether two pillows or flat is more comfortable for client or elevate the head of the bed 30 degrees. Turn at least every 2 hours to encourage secretion drainage. Consider maneuvers to drain areas of lungs with retained secretions by gravity if tolerated by client. If unilateral reexpansion is needed, have client lie with side requiring expansion up: "good side down, affected lung up."

Nurse Alert: Specific positioning may be ordered after some types of thoracic surgery.

3. Controlled coughing
   a. Place client in upright position. High Fowler's leaning forward, or with knees bent and a small pillow or hand to support the abdomen may augment expiratory pressure.   ____ ____ ____ _____
   b. Instruct client to take two slow, deep breaths, inhaling through the nose and exhaling out the mouth.   ____ ____ ____ _____
   c. Instruct client to inhale deeply a third time, hold this breath, and count to three; then cough deeply for two or three consecutive coughs without inhaling between coughs. Instruct the client to push air forcefully out of the lungs.   ____ ____ ____ _____

4. Provide assistive equipment.
   a. Apply CPAP/BiPAP.
      (1) Position client.
      (2) Position face mask or nasal mask tightly and adjust head strap until seal is maintained and client is able to tolerate.   ____ ____ ____ _____
      (3) Instruct client to breathe normally.   ____ ____ ____ _____
      (4) Apply at ordered setting for prescribed length of time.   ____ ____ ____ _____
   b. Obtain PEFR measurements.
      (1) Instruct client about purpose and rationale.   ____ ____ ____ _____
      (2) Place client in an upright position.   ____ ____ ____ _____
      (3) Slide mouthpiece into base of the numbered scale.   ____ ____ ____ _____
      (4) Instruct client to take a deep breath.   ____ ____ ____ _____
      (5) Have client place meter mouthpiece in the mouth and close lips, making a firm seal.   ____ ____ ____ _____
      (6) Have client blow out as hard and fast as possible through the mouth only.   ____ ____ ____ _____
      (7) This maneuver should be repeated two additional times, with the highest number recorded.   ____ ____ ____ _____
      (8) If client is to record PEFR at home, have client demonstrate PEFR technique independently and assess ability to record PEFR accurately in a diary.   ____ ____ ____ _____

5. Use Completion Protocol.   ____ ____ ____ _____

Evaluation

1. Observe client's body alignment and position whenever in visual contact with client. Reposition as needed, at least every 2 hours.   ____ ____ ____ _____

	S	U	NP	Comments

2. Auscultate lungs for adventitious sounds. ____ ____ ____ _____

3. Monitor client's respiratory status. ____ ____ ____ _____

4. Monitor ABGs/pulse oximetry. ____ ____ ____ _____

5. Observe technique of client/family using equipment. ____ ____ ____ _____

6. Observe return demonstration from client/family member with PEFR. ____ ____ ____ _____

7. Determine client's PEFR and compare with prior best. ____ ____ ____ _____

8. Ask client to explain purpose and benefits of positioning and therapies. ____ ____ ____ _____

- Identify unexpected outcomes and intervene as necessary. ____ ____ ____ _____

- Record and report intervention and client's response. ____ ____ ____ _____

Name _____Hien Dang_____ Date _1/31/08_ Instructor's Name _Babot, RN_

Performance Checklist: Skill 31.3

Airway Management: Suctioning

	S	U	NP	Comments

Assessment

1. Observe for signs and symptoms of excess secretions in the oral cavity and productive cough without expectoration. ✓

2. Assess for airway obstruction. ✓

3. Assess for risk factors for need for suctioning. ✓

4. Assess client's understanding of procedure. ✓

Implementation

1. Use Standard Protocol. ✓

2. Position client. Prepare suction kit/catheter. ✓

3. Apply gloves. Preparation for all types of suctioning.
   a. Fill basin or cup with approximately 100 ml of water. ✓
   b. Connect one end of connecting tubing to suction machine. Check that equipment is functioning properly by suctioning a small amount of water from basin. ✓
   c. Turn suction device on. Set regulator to appropriate negative pressure: wall suction, 80 to 120 mm Hg; portable suction, 7 to 15 mm Hg for adults. ✓

4. Oropharyngeal suctioning
   a. Consider applying mask or face shield. Attach suction catheter to connecting tubing. Remove oxygen mask if present.
   b. Insert catheter into client's mouth. With suction applied, move catheter around mouth, including pharynx and gum line, until secretions are cleared. ✓
   c. Encourage client to cough, and repeat suctioning if needed. Replace oxygen mask if used. ✓
   d. Suction water from basin through catheter until catheter is cleared of secretions. ✓
   e. Place catheter in a clean, dry area for

	S	U	NP	Comments

reuse with suction turned off or within client's reach, with suction on, if client is capable of suctioning self. √ ___ ___ _____

f. Discard water if not used by client. Clean basin or dispose of cup. Remove gloves and dispose. √ ___ ___ _____

5. Nasotracheal suctioning
   a. Apply one sterile glove to each hand, or apply nonsterile glove to nondominant hand and sterile glove to dominant hand. Attach nonsterile suction tubing to sterile catheter, keeping the hand holding catheter sterile. √ ___ ___ _____

   b. Secure catheter to tubing aseptically. Coat distal 6 to 8 cm (2-3 inches) of catheter with water-soluble lubricants. √ ___ ___ _____

   c. Remove oxygen delivery device, if present, with nondominant hand. Use dominant hand to insert catheter into nares during inspiration without applying suction. Do not force catheter. √ ___ ___ _____

Nurse Alert: Keep oxygen delivery device readily available.

   d. Advance catheter to just above entrance into trachea. Allow client to take a breath. √ ___ ___ _____

   e. Insert catheter approximately 16 cm (6 to 8 inches) in adults. Advance catheter until resistance is felt or client coughs. √ ___ ___ _____

   f. Apply intermittent suction by placing and releasing nondominant thumb and forefinger, over vent of catheter, and slowly withdraw catheter while rotating it back and forth between thumb and forefinger. The maximum time catheter may remain in airway is 10 seconds. Encourage client to cough. √ ___ ___ _____

Nurse Alert: If catheter grabs mucosa, release suction.

   g. Rinse catheter and connecting tubing by suctioning water from the basin until tubing is clear. Dispose of catheter and remaining saline in basin. Turn off suction device. √ ___ ___ _____

6. Endotracheal or tracheostomy tube suctioning
   a. Apply one sterile glove to each hand, or apply nonsterile glove to nondominant hand and sterile glove to dominant hand. Attach nonsterile suction tubing to sterile catheter, keeping hand holding catheter sterile. √ ___ ___ _____

	S	U	NP	Comments

b. Check that equipment is functioning properly by suctioning small amounts of saline from basin. ✓

c. Hyperoxygenate client before suctioning, using manual resuscitation bag or sigh mechanism on mechanical ventilator. ✓

d. Open swivel adapter, or, if necessary, remove oxygen or humidity delivery device with nondominant hand. ✓

e. Without applying suction and using dominant thumb and forefinger, gently but quickly insert catheter into artificial airway (best to time catheter insertion with inspiration) until resistance is met or client coughs, then pull back 1 cm. ✓

f. Apply intermittent suction by placing and releasing nondominant thumb over vent of catheter and slowly withdraw catheter while rotating it. Maximum time in airway is 10 seconds. Encourage client to cough. ✓

g. Close swivel adapter or replace oxygen delivery device. Encourage client to deep breathe. Some clients respond well to several manual breaths from the mechanical ventilator or resuscitation bag. ✓

h. Rinse catheter and connecting tube with NS until clear. Use continuous suction. ✓

i. Assess client's cardiopulmonary status for secretion clearance and complications. Repeat secretions. Allow adequate time (at least 1 full minute) between suction passes for ventilation and reoxygenation. ✓

j. Perform nasopharyngeal and oropharyngeal suctioning to clear upper airway of secretions. After these suctionings are performed, catheter is contaminated; do not reinsert into endotracheal tube (ET) or tracheostomy tube. ✓

k. Disconnect catheter from connecting tube. Roll catheter around fingers of dominant hand. Pull glove off inside out so that catheter remains in glove. Pull off other glove in same way. Discard into appropriate receptacle. Turn off suction device. ✓

l. Place unopened suction kit on suction machine or at head of bed. ✓

7. ET or tracheostomy tube suctioning with a closed-system (in-line) catheter
   a. Attach suction.

	S	U	NP	Comments

(1) In many institutions, catheter is attached to mechanical ventilator circuit by personnel from respiratory therapy. If not already in place, open suction catheter package using aseptic technique, attach closed-suction catheter to ventilator circuit by removing swivel adapter and placing closed-suction catheter apparatus on ET or tracheostomy tube, and connect Y on mechanical ventilator circuit to closed-suction catheter with flex tubing.

(2) Connect one end of connecting tube to suction machine and connect other to end of closed-system or in-line suction catheter if not already done. Turn suction device on and set vacuum regulator to appropriate negative pressure (80-120 mm Hg for adults).

b. Hyperinflate/hyperoxygenate client.

c. Unlock suction control mechanism if required by manufacturer. Open saline port and attach saline syringe or vial.

d. Pick up suction catheter enclosed in plastic sleeve with dominant hand. Open saline port and attach saline syringe or vial.

e. Wait until client inhales NS or mechanical ventilator delivers a breath to dispense NS, then quickly but gently insert catheter on next inhalation. To insert catheter, use a repeating maneuver of pushing catheter and sliding (or pulling) plastic back between thumb and forefinger until resistance is felt or client coughs.

f. Encourage client to cough and apply suction by squeezing on mechanism while withdrawing. Be sure to withdraw catheter completely into plastic sheath so it does not obstruct airflow.

g. Reassess cardiopulmonary status, including pulse oximetry, to determine need for subsequent suctioning or complications. Repeat steps c through f one or two more times to clear secretions. Allow at least 1 full minute between suction passes for ventilation and reoxygenation.

	S	U	NP	Comments

h. When airway is clear, withdraw catheter completely into sheath. Be sure black line on catheter is visible in sheath. Squeeze vial or push syringe while applying suction to rinse inner lumen of catheter. Use at least 5 to 10 ml of NS. Lock suction mechanism, if applicable, and turn off suction. ✓ _____ _____ _____

i. Client may require suctioning of oral cavity. ✓ _____ _____ _____

8. Use Completion Protocol. ✓ _____ _____ _____

Evaluation

1. Auscultate lungs and compare client's respiratory assessments before and after suctioning. ✓ _____ _____ _____

2. Ask client if breathing is easier and if congestion is decreased. ✓ _____ _____ _____

3. Observe client's respirations. ✓ _____ _____ _____

4. Observe client's technique and compliance with suctioning procedures. ✓ _____ _____ _____

• Identify unexpected outcomes and intervene as necessary. ✓ _____ _____ _____

• Record and report intervention and client's response. ✓ _____ _____ _____

Name _____ Date _____ Instructor's Name _____

Performance Checklist: Skill 31.4

Airway Management: Endotracheal Tube and Tracheostomy Care

	S	U	NP	Comments

Assessment

1. Assess client for signs and symptoms indicating the need to perform care of the artificial airway. _____ _____ _____ _____

2. Identify factors that increase risk of complications from artificial airways. _____ _____ _____ _____

3. Auscultate lungs. _____ _____ _____ _____

4. Assess client's knowledge and comfort with procedure. _____ _____ _____ _____

5. If applicable, assess client's understanding of and ability to perform own tracheostomy care. _____ _____ _____ _____

Implementation

1. Use Standard Protocol. _____ _____ _____ _____

2. Endotracheal tube care
   a. Initiate suction. _____ _____ _____ _____

Nurse Alert: An oral airway should be immediately accessible in the event the client bites down and obstructs the ET tube.

   b. Leave Yankauer suction catheter connected to suction source. _____ _____ _____ _____
   c. Prepare tape. Cut piece of tape long enough to go completely around client's head from naris to naris plus 15 cm (6 inches)—about 30-60 cm (1–2 feet). Lay adhesive side up on bedside table. Cut and lay 8 to 16 cm (3-6 inches) of tape, adhesive side down, in center of long strip to prevent tape from sticking to hair. _____ _____ _____ _____
   d. Apply gloves. Have an assistant also apply a pair of gloves and hold ET tube firmly so that tube does not move. _____ _____ _____ _____
   e. Carefully remove tape from ET tube and client's face. If tape is difficult to remove, moisten with water or adhesive tape

remover. Discard tape in appropriate receptacle if nearby. If not, place soiled tape on bedside table or on distant end of towel.

f. Use adhesive remover swab to remove excess adhesive left on face after tape removal.

g. Remove oral airway or bite block if present.

h. Clean mouth, gums, and teeth opposite ET tube with mouthwash solution and 4×4 gauze, sponge-tipped applicators, or saline swabs. Brush teeth as indicated. If necessary, administer oropharyngeal suctioning with Yankauer catheter.

i. Oral ET tube only: Note "cm" ET tube marking at lips or gums. With help of assistant, move ET tube to opposite side or center of mouth. Do not change tube depth.

j. Repeat oral cleaning as in step h on opposite side of mouth.

k. Clean face and neck with soapy washcloth; rinse and dry. Shave male client as necessary.

l. Pour small amount of tincture of benzoin on clean 2×2 gauze and dot on upper lip (oral ET tube) or across nose (nasal ET tube) and cheeks to ear. Allow to dry completely.

m. Slip tape under client's head and neck, adhesive side down. Take care not to twist tape or catch hair. Do not allow tape to stick to itself. It helps to stick tape gently to tongue blade, which serves as a guide. Then slide tongue blade under client's neck. Center tape so that double-faced tape extends around back of neck from ear to ear.

n. On one side of face, secure tape from ear to naris (nasal ET tube) or edge of mouth (oral ET tube). Tear remaining tape in half lengthwise, forming two pieces that are $\frac{1}{2}$ to $\frac{3}{4}$ inch wide. Secure bottom half of tape across upper lip (oral ET tube) or across top of nose (nasal ET tube). Wrap top half of tape around tube.

o. Gently pull other side of tape firmly to pick up slack and secure to remaining side of face. Assistant can release hold when tube is secure. Nurse may want assistant to help reinsert oral airway.

p. Clean oral airway in warm soapy water and rinse well. Hydrogen peroxide can

	S	U	NP	Comments

aid in removal of crusted secretions.
Shake excess water from oral airway.

q. Reinsert oral airway without pushing
tongue into oropharynx.

3. Tracheostomy care

a. Suction tracheostomy. Before removing
gloves, remove soiled trach dressing and
discard in glove with coiled catheter.

b. While client is replenishing oxygen stores,
prepare equipment on bedside table.
Open sterile trach kit. Open three 4×4
gauze packages using aseptic technique
and pour NS on one package and
hydrogen peroxide on another. Leave
third package dry.

c. Open two cotton-tipped swabbed
packages and pour NS on one package
and hydrogen peroxide on the other.

d. Open sterile trach package. Unwrap
sterile basin and pour about 2 cm
(¾ inch) hydrogen peroxide into it.
Open small sterile brush package and
place aseptically into sterile basin.

e. If using large roll of twill tape, cut
appropriate length of tape and lay aside
in dry area. Do not recap hydrogen
peroxide and NS.

f. Apply gloves. Keep dominant hand
sterile throughout procedure.

g. Remove oxygen source.

**Nurse Alert: It is important to stabilize the
tracheostomy tube at all times to prevent injury
and discomfort.**

h. If a nondisposable inner cannula is used:
(1) Remove with nondominant hand.
Drop inner cannula into hydrogen
peroxide basin.

(2) Place trach collar or T tube and
ventilator oxygen source over or
near outer cannula.

(3) To prevent oxygen desaturation in
affected clients, quickly pick up
inner cannula and use small brush to
remove secretions inside and outside
cannula.

(4) Hold inner cannula over basin and
rinse with normal saline (NS), using
nondominant hand to pour.

(5) Replace inner cannula and secure
"locking" mechanism. Reapply
ventilator or oxygen sources.

i. If a disposable inner cannula is used:
  (1) Remove cannula from manufacturer's packaging.

_____ _____ _____ _____

  (2) Withdraw inner cannula and replace with new cannula. Lock into position.

_____ _____ _____ _____

  (3) Dispose of contaminated cannula in appropriate receptacle.

_____ _____ _____ _____

j. Using hydrogen peroxide–prepared cotton-tipped swabs and 4 × 4 gauze, clean exposed outer cannula surfaces and stoma under faceplate, extending 5 to 10 cm (2-4 inches) in all directions from stoma. Clean in circular motion from stoma site outward, using dominant hand to handle sterile supplies.

_____ _____ _____ _____

k. Using NS-prepared cotton-tipped swabs and 4 × 4 gauze, rinse hydrogen peroxide from trach tube and skin surfaces.

_____ _____ _____ _____

l. Using dry 4 × 4 gauze, pat lightly at skin and exposed outer cannula surfaces.

_____ _____ _____ _____

m. Instruct assistant, if available, to hold trach tube securely in place while ties are cut.

_____ _____ _____ _____

Nurse Alert: Trach tube must be held continuously to prevent accidental extubation.

  (1) Cut length of twill tape long enough to go around client's neck two times, about 60 to 75 cm (24-30 inches) for an adult. Cut ends on a diagonal.

_____ _____ _____ _____

Nurse Alert: Secure trach ties with one finger slack. For accidental extubation, call for assistance and manually ventilate client with bag-in-mask, if necessary. Tracheostomy obturator should be kept at bedside with fresh tracheostomy to facilitate reinsertion of the outer cannula, if dislodged.

  (2) Insert one end of tie through faceplate eyelet and pull ends even.

_____ _____ _____ _____

  (3) Slide both ends of tie behind head and around neck to other eyelet, and insert one tie through second eyelet.

_____ _____ _____ _____

  (4) Pull snugly.

_____ _____ _____ _____

  (5) Tie ends securely in double square knot, allowing space for only one finger in tie.

_____ _____ _____ _____

n. Insert fresh trach dressing under clean ties and faceplate.

_____ _____ _____ _____

o. Position client comfortably and assess respiratory status.

_____ _____ _____ _____

4. Use Completion Protocol.

_____ _____ _____ _____

	S	U	NP	Comments

Evaluation

1. Auscultate lungs. Observe position of airway, oral mucosa, vital signs, and equal bilateral breath sounds. _____ _____ _____ _____

2. Monitor client for fever and stoma for infection. _____ _____ _____ _____

3. Compare assessments made before and after artificial airway care. Observe for tissue breakdown or persistent dried secretions. _____ _____ _____ _____

4. Observe client's ability to perform trach care. _____ _____ _____ _____

• Identify unexpected outcomes and intervene as necessary. _____ _____ _____ _____

• Record and report intervention and client's response. _____ _____ _____ _____

Performance Checklist: Skill 31.5

Managing Closed Chest Drainage Systems (Including Managing Postoperative Autotransfusions)

	S	U	NP	Comments

Assessment

1. Perform a complete respiratory assessment.

2. Observe for changes from initial assessment.

3. Ask if client is able to breathe deeply and comfortably.

4. Review laboratory results.

Implementation

1. Use Standard Protocol.

2. Set up water-seal system.
   a. Obtain a chest drainage system. Remove wrappers and prepare to set up as a two- or three-chamber system.
   b. While maintaining sterility of the drainage tubing, stand system upright and add sterile water or NS to appropriate compartments.
   c. For a two-chamber system (without suction), add sterile solution to water-seal chamber (second chamber), bringing fluid to the required level as indicated.
   d. For a three-chamber system (without suction), add sterile solution to the water-seal chamber (second chamber). Add amount of sterile solution prescribed by physician to the suction control (third) chamber, usually 20 cm (8 inches). Connect tubing from suction control chamber to suction source.

3. Set up waterless system.
   a. Remove sterile wrappers and prepare to set up.
   b. For a two-chamber system (without suction), nothing is added or needs to be done to system.
   c. For a three-chamber waterless system with suction, connect tubing from suction control chamber to suction source.

d. Instill 15 ml sterile water or NS into diagnostic indicator injection port located on top of system.

4. Tape all connections in a spiral fashion using 1-inch adhesive tape. Then check both systems for patency.

a. Clamp from drainage tubing that will connect client to system.
b. Connect tubing from float ball chamber to suction source.

Nurse Alert: Bubbling should stop after a short time in the absence of an air leak. If bubbling continues, check all connections.

c. Turn on suction to prescribed level.

5. Turn off suction source and unclamp drainage tubing before connecting client to system.

6. Position the client.
a. Use semi-Fowler's to high Fowler's position to evacuate air (pneumothorax).
b. Use high Fowler's position to drain fluid (hemothorax).

7. Assist physician with chest tube insertion by providing equipment and analgesic and offering support and instruction to the client.

8. Apply gloves. Help physician attach drainage tube to chest tube.

9. Tape tube connection between chest and drainage tubes.

10. Check patency of air vents in system.
a. Make sure water-seal vent has no occlusion.
b. Check that suction control chamber vent has no occlusion when using suction.
c. Know that waterless systems have relief valves without caps.

11. Coil excess tubing on mattress next to client. Secure with a rubber band and safety pin or system's clamp.

12. Adjust tubing to hang in a straight line from top of mattress to drainage chamber.

13. Provide two shodded hemostats for each chest tube. Attach shodded hemostats to top of client's bed with adhesive tape or clamp to client's clothing during ambulation.

14. Care for client with chest tube(s).
  a. Monitor vital signs, oxygen saturation, skin color, breath sounds, rate, depth, and ease of respirations, drainage, and insertion site every 15 minutes for first 2 hours.

   ____ ____ ____ _____

  b. Monitor color, consistency, and amount of drainage every 15 minutes for first 2 hours. Mark time and level of drainage on calibrated write-on periodically. Indicate date and time that drainage was first collected on drainage chamber's write-on surface.

   ____ ____ ____ _____

  c. Observe chest dressing for drainage.
  d. Palpate around tube for swelling and crepitus (crackling sound).

   ____ ____ ____ _____

  e. Check that tubing is free of kinks and dependent loops.

   ____ ____ ____ _____

  f. Observe for fluctuation of drainage in tubing with inspiration or expiration.

   ____ ____ ____ _____

  g. Keep system upright and below level of chest.

   ____ ____ ____ _____

  h. Observe and check for leaks by constant bubbling in water-seal chamber (intermittent bubbling with expiration is normal). Check for fluctuation with client's inspiration and expiration.

   ____ ____ ____ _____

15. Obtain specimen.
  a. Apply gloves. Cleanse resealing diaphragm or tubing with an antiseptic.

   ____ ____ ____ _____

  b. Insert needle with bevel in the fresh drainage.

   ____ ____ ____ _____

  c. Gently aspirate appropriate amount of fluid and place into properly labeled container.

   ____ ____ ____ _____

  d. Recleanse diaphragm with antiseptic swab.

   ____ ____ ____ _____

16. Assist in chest tube removal.
  a. Administer prescribed medication for pain relief about 30 minutes before procedure.

   ____ ____ ____ _____

  b. Assist client to sit on edge of bed or to lie on side without chest tubes.

   ____ ____ ____ _____

  c. Physician prepares an occlusive dressing of petrolatum gauze on a pressure dressing and sets it aside on a sterile field.

   ____ ____ ____ _____

  d. Physician asks client to take a deep breath and hold it or exhale completely and hold it.
  e. Physician quickly pulls out chest tube.

   ____ ____ ____ _____

  f. Physician quickly applies prepared dressing over wound and firmly secures it in position with elastic bandage

   369

(Elastoplast) or wide tape. Physician
sometimes uses skin clips or draws purse
string sutures together before applying
dressing.

17. Perform postoperative autotransfusion.
   a. Set up the Pleur-evac autotransfusion
     system (ATS).
   b. Make sure all connections are tight and
     all clamps are open.
   c. A 200 μ double-sided mesh filter is
     located in the ATS bag to filter drainage.
   d. ATS collection bag has a capacity of
     1000 ml, marked increments of 25 ml,
     and an area for marking times and
     amounts.
   e. Continue collection.
     (1) Open Pleur-evac A-1500
        replacement bag using proper
        technique and close two white
        clamps.
     (2) Use high-negativity relief valve to
        reduce excessive negativity.
     (3) Perform bag transfer.
        (a) Close clamp on chest drainage
           tubing.
        (b) Close two white clamps on top
           of initial ATS collection bag.
        (c) Connect chest drainage tube to
           new ATS bag using red
           containers. Make certain that
           all connections are tight.
        (d) Open all clamps on chest
           drainage tube and replacement
           bag.
   f. Connect red and blue connectors on top
     of initial collection bag, and remove it
     by lifting it from side hook and then
     from foot hook.
   g. Secure replacement bag by connecting
     foot hook, replacing metal frame into
     side hook of Pleur-evac unit, and
     pushing down to secure frame into
     hook.
   h. Replacement bag is removed by placing
     the thumbs on top of metal frame and
     pushing up with fingers to slide bag out.
   i. Initiate Pleur-evac autotransfusion
     reinfusion.
     (1) Use a new microaggregate filter to
        reinfuse each autotransfusion bag.
     (2) Access bag by inverting it, spiking it

	S	U	NP	Comments

through spike port with microaggregate filter, and twisting.

(3) With bag upside down, gently squeeze it to remove the air and prime the filter with blood.

(4) Hang bag on an intravenous (IV) pole and continue to prime tubing until all air is gone. Clamp tubing, attach it to client's IV access, and adjust clamp to deliver the reinfusion at the appropriate rate.

(5) If ordered, anticoagulants can be added to the reinfusion through self-sealing port in autotransfusion connector.

j. Discontinue autotransfusion.

(1) Clamp chest drainage tube and connect it directly to Pleur-evac unit using red and blue connectors.

(2) Open chest drainage tube clamp.

Nurse Alert: Stripping or milking the chest tube is controversial. Refer to aging policy.

18. Use Completion Protocol.

Evaluation

1. Monitor client's respiratory status, oxygen saturation, and chest pain.

2. Auscultate lungs and observe chest expansion.

3. Monitor vital signs and H&H.

4. Monitor ability to use deep breathing exercises.

5. Evaluate client's level of comfort.

6. Monitor continued functioning of system, as indicated by reduction in the amount of drainage, resolution of the air leak, and complete reexpansion of the lung.

7. Monitor client's oxygen saturation.

• Identify unexpected outcomes and intervene as necessary.

• Record and report intervention and client's response.

Performance Checklist: Skill 32.1

Inserting Nasogastric Tube (Includes Checking Placement of Nasal Tube)

	S	U	NP	Comments

Assessment

1. Ask client about history of nasal surgery or trauma. Assess client's nares and oral cavity for deviated nasal septum, nasal surgery, inability to breathe well when either nasal opening is occluded, and nasal or oral irritation or bleeding.

2. Palpate client's abdomen for distention or pain and auscultate for bowel sounds.

3. Determine whether client had NG tube insertion in the past.

4. Assess client's level of consciousness and ability to cooperate or assist with the procedure.

5. Check medical record for surgeon's order, type of nasogastric (NG) tube to be placed, and whether tube is to attach to suction or drainage bag.

Implementation

1. Use Standard Protocol.

Nurse Alert: Have suction equipment and emesis basin within reach.

2. Prepare equipment at bedside. Cut a piece of tape about 4 inches (10 cm) long, and split one half of it into two pieces to form a Y.

3. Place client in high Fowler's position with pillows behind the head and shoulders.

4. Place towel over client's chest and provide tissues to client.

5. Instruct client to relax and breathe normally while occluding one naris. Repeat with other naris and select side with best airflow.

6. Apply gloves. Stand on client's right side if right-handed, left side if left-handed.

	S	U	NP	Comments

7. Measure estimated length of tube to reach well into stomach.
   a. Measure distance from tip of nose to earlobe to xiphoid process of sternum. _____ _____ _____ _____
   b. Mark a 50 cm (20 inches) point on the tube, then perform the traditional measurement. Insertion point should be midway between the markings. _____ _____ _____ _____

8. Mark this distance on tube with a removable piece of tape or an indelible marker. _____ _____ _____ _____

9. Curve 10 to 15 cm (4 to 6 inches) of end of tube tightly around index finger and then release. _____ _____ _____ _____

10. Lubricate about 10 cm (4 inches) of the distal end of the tube with a water-soluble lubricant. _____ _____ _____ _____

11. Tell client that insertion is about to begin, and ask client to extend neck back against pillow. _____ _____ _____ _____

12. Insert tube slowly through naris with curved end pointing downward. Continue to insert tube along floor of nasal passage, aiming down toward ear. If resistance is met, apply gentle downward pressure to advance tube. _____ _____ _____ _____

13. If resistance is met, try to rotate the tube. With continued resistance, withdraw tube, allow client to rest, lubricate it again, and attempt insertion in opposite nostril. _____ _____ _____ _____

Nurse Alert: Do not force, which may cause trauma to tissues. If unable to insert tube in either naris, stop procedure and notify physician.

14. Insert tube to nasopharynx, rotate it toward the opposite nostril, then pass just above oropharynx.
   a. Stop and allow client to relax. Provide tissues as needed _____ _____ _____ _____
   b. Explain that the next step requires client to swallow. Give client glass of water, unless contraindicated. _____ _____ _____ _____

15. Ask client to bend head forward and swallow small sips of water if allowed or to swallow without water as tube is advanced. Advance tube 1 to 2 inches (2.5 to 5 cm) with each swallow. If coughing or gagging occurs, withdraw tube a bit and allow client to relax and breathe easily. _____ _____ _____ _____

Nurse Alert: If vomiting occurs, assist client in clearing airway. Oral suctioning may be needed. Do not proceed until airway is cleared.

374

	S	U	NP	Comments

16. Ask client whether tube feels as though it is coiling in back of throat, and check back of oropharynx using tongue blade to compress client's tongue. If tube has coiled, withdraw it until the tip is back in the oropharynx. Then reinsert with client swallowing. ___ ___ ___ _____

17. Continue to advance tube with swallowing until tape or mark is reached. Temporarily anchor tube to cheek with a piece of tape until placement is checked. ___ ___ ___ _____

18. Verify tube placement.
    a. Ask client to speak. ___ ___ ___ _____
    b. Inspect posterior pharynx for presence of coiled tube. ___ ___ ___ _____
    c. Attach catheter-tipped syringe to end of tube, then aspirate gently back on syringe to obtain gastric contents, observing color. ___ ___ ___ _____
    d. Measure pH of aspirate with the color-coded pH paper with range of whole numbers at least 1 to 11. ___ ___ ___ _____

Nurse Alert: Be sure to use Gastrocult and not Hemoccult test.

19. If pH of aspirate is not 4 or less, advance tube by about 2.5 to 5 cm (1-2 inches) and repeat steps a through d. ___ ___ ___ _____

20. Anchor tube to nose.
    a. After tube is inserted and position verified, clamp tube or connect to drainage bag or suction. ___ ___ ___ _____
    b. Tape tube to nose. ___ ___ ___ _____
       (1) Apply tincture of benzoin sparingly to nose and allow it to become "tacky." ___ ___ ___ _____
       (2) Wrap two ends of tape around tube. ___ ___ ___ _____
       (3) Apply tube fixation device using shaped adhesive patch. ___ ___ ___ _____
    c. Fasten rubber band to end of NG tube in a slip knot, and pin rubber band to client's gown, allowing enough slack for movement of head. ___ ___ ___ _____
    d. Keep head of bed elevated at least 30 degrees unless physician orders otherwise. ___ ___ ___ _____
    e. Remove gloves and wash hands. ___ ___ ___ _____

21. Once placement is confirmed:
    a. Place a mark or tape on the point where the tube exits the client's nose. ___ ___ ___ _____
    b. Measure length from the mark to the connector. ___ ___ ___ _____
    c. Document findings from steps a and b. ___ ___ ___ _____

	S	U	NP	Comments

22. Provide regular oral hygiene every 2 to 3 hours.

____ ____ ____ _____

23. Use Completion Protocol.

____ ____ ____ _____

Evaluation

1. Auscultate bowel sounds. Palpate client's abdomen for distention and pain.

____ ____ ____ _____

2. Evaluate client's level of comfort.

____ ____ ____ _____

3. Observe color of drainage and patency of tube.

____ ____ ____ _____

4. Observe client's oral and nasal mucosa.

____ ____ ____ _____

• Identify unexpected outcomes and intervene as necessary.

____ ____ ____ _____

• Record and report intervention and client's response.

____ ____ ____ _____

Name _____ Date _____ Instructor's Name _____

Performance Checklist: Skill 32.2

Irrigating Nasogastric Tube

	S	U	NP	Comments

Assessment

1. Assess the volume, color, and character of gastric secretions.

2. Assess client's abdomen for abdomen for distention or pain.

3. Assess bowel sounds and passage of flatus.

Implementation

1. Use Standard Protocol.

2. Apply gloves. Verify tube placement.

3. Draw up 30 ml of normal saline solution into large syringe.

4. Pinch or clamp NG tube and remove from suction source. Lay end of suction tubing on towel.

Nurse Alert: Do not introduce saline through air vent on Salem sump tube.

5. Insert tip of irrigation syringe into end of NG tube and unkink tubing. Inject saline solution steadily; do not force.

6. If unable to instill fluid, check for kinks in tubing, reposition client on left side, and try again. Report repeated resistance.

7. When saline solution has been instilled, withdraw fluid by pulling back gently on syringe. Record difference in volume instilled and volume withdrawn. If equal, no documentation is required.

8. Reconnect NG tube to suction. Remove and discard gloves and wash hands.

9. Use Completion Protocol.

Evaluation

1. Palpate the client's abdomen for distention and pain.

	S	U	NP	Comments

2. Auscultate bowel sounds. ____ ____ ____ _____

3. Measure amount and characteristics of NG secretions. ____ ____ ____ _____

4. Verify correct position of tube.

5. Evaluate client's comfort level. ____ ____ ____ _____

• Identify unexpected outcomes and intervene as necessary. ____ ____ ____ _____

• Record and report intervention and client's response. ____ ____ ____ _____

Performance Checklist: Skill 32.3

Removing Nasogastric Tube

	S	U	NP	Comments

Assessment

1. Palpate for pain or abdominal distention. ___ ___ ___ _____

2. Ask client about nausea or abdominal pain. ___ ___ ___ _____

3. Assess for signs of returning bowel function, such as bowel movements, flatus, and presence of bowel. ___ ___ ___ _____

Implementation

1. Use Standard Protocol. ___ ___ ___ _____

2. Verify physician's order. ___ ___ ___ _____

3. Place towel over client's chest to protect gown and cover tube. ___ ___ ___ _____

4. Apply gloves. Turn off suction and disconnect NG tube from drainage bag or suction. Remove tape or fixation device from client's nose and unpin tube from gown. ___ ___ ___ _____

5. Stand on appropriate side for use of dominant hand. ___ ___ ___ _____

6. Attach large syringe to tube and flush with 20 ml of air. ___ ___ ___ _____

7. Hand client facial tissue and ask client to take a deep breath and hold it as tube is removed. ___ ___ ___ _____

8. Tell client that removal of tube is about to begin and will not be as uncomfortable as insertion. ___ ___ ___ _____

9. Clamp or kink tube securely and pull tube out quickly and steadily onto towel. ___ ___ ___ _____

10. Measure volume of drainage and note character of content. Record on I&O summary. Dispose of NG tube. Remove and discard gloves and wash hands. ___ ___ ___ _____

11. Clean nares and provide mouth care. ___ ___ ___ _____

12. Use Completion Protocol. ___ ___ ___ _____

Evaluation

1. Determine client's comfort level after tube removal and mouth care.

   ___ ___ ___ _____

2. Palpate client's abdomen and auscultate for bowel sounds.

   ___ ___ ___ _____

- Identify unexpected outcomes and intervene as necessary.

   ___ ___ ___ _____

- Record and report intervention and client's response.

   ___ ___ ___ _____

Name _____ Date _____ Instructor's Name _____

Performance Checklist: Skill 34.1

Removing Fecal Impactions

	S	U	NP	Comments

Assessment

1. Assess client's normal and current bowel elimination pattern.

2. Assess client's abdomen for distention, auscultate for the presence of bowel sounds, and palpate the abdomen for masses.

3. Auscultate for bowel sounds.

4. Observe pattern and consistency of stool.

5. Measure client's current vital signs to establish a baseline.

6. Determine whether client is receiving anticoagulants.

7. Check client's record for physician's order for digital removal of impaction.

Implementation

1. Use Standard Protocol.

2. Apply gloves. Assist client to left side-lying position with knees flexed.

3. Drape client's trunk and lower extremities with bath blanket and place waterproof pad under buttocks.

4. Place bedpan next to client.

5. Lubricate gloved index finger with lubricating jelly.

Nurse Alert: Observe for the presence of irritation to perianal skin.

6. Insert index finger into rectum.

7. Gradually advance finger slowly along rectal wall toward umbilicus.

8. Gently loosen fecal mass by massaging around it. Work finger into hardened mass.

9. Work stool downward toward end of rectum. Remove small sections of feces.

	S	U	NP	Comments

10. Periodically assess heart rate and look for signs of fatigue.

Nurse Alert: Stop procedure if heart rate drops or rhythm changes or if bleeding occurs.

11. Continue to clear rectum of feces and allow client to rest at intervals.

12. After removal of impaction, provide washcloth and towel to wash buttocks and anal area.

13. Remove bedpan and dispose of feces. Remove gloves by turning inside out and discarding in proper receptacle.

14. Assist client to toilet or clean bedpan.

15. Use Completion Protocol.

Evaluation

1. Perform rectal examination for stool. Palpate abdomen.

2. Reassess vital signs and compare to baseline values.

3. Auscultate bowel sounds.

4. Palpate abdomen for tenderness.

5. Monitor bowel elimination patterns.

• Identify unexpected outcomes and intervene as necessary.

• Record and report intervention and client's response.

Performance Checklist: Skill 34.2

Pouching an Enterostomy

	S	U	NP	Comments

Assessment

1. Identify the type of ostomy.

2. Auscultate for bowel sounds.

3. Observe skin barrier and pouch for leakage and length of time in place.

4. Assess client's periostomal skin condition.

5. Assess client's stoma for size, shape, type, color, and drainage.

Nurse Alert: Intact skin barriers with no evidence of leakage do not need to be changed daily.

Implementation

1. Use Standard Protocol.

2. Apply gloves. Inspect pouch periodically to see if it has to be emptied. Empty when one-third to one-half full.

3. Place towel or waterproof barrier under client.

4. Apply gloves. Remove used pouch and skin barrier gently by pushing down on the skin and lifting up on the barrier. An adhesive remover may be needed.

5. Cleanse periostomal skin gently with warm tap water using gauze pads or clean washcloth. Do not scrub skin. Allow to dry completely.

Nurse Alert: Bleeding into pouch is abnormal.

6. Measure stoma for correct size of pouching system.

7. Select appropriate pouch for client. For a custom fit pouch, use an ostomy guide to cut opening on the pouch $1/16$ to $1/8$ inch larger than stoma before removing backing. Barrier of flange for two-piece appliance should be at least $1/4$ inch larger than the

stoma. Prepare pouch by removing backing from barrier and adhesive.

____ ____ ____ _____

Nurse Alert: The stoma should be measured at each pouching system change to determine the correct size of the equipment. Follow manufacturer's directions and measuring guide to determine size of pouch to use.

8. Apply thin circle of barrier paste around opening in pouch; allow to dry.

____ ____ ____ _____

Nurse Alert: The skin barrier may need to be trimmed if the stoma location is close to a client's abdominal incision.

9. Apply skin barrier and pouch. Use barrier paste to fill in creases next to stoma. Let dry 1 to 2 minutes.

____ ____ ____ _____

   a. For one-piece system:
     (1) Use skin sealant wipes on skin directly under the adhesive skin barrier or pouch; allow to dry. Starting from the bottom and working up and around the sides, press adhesive backing of pouch and/or skin barrier smoothly against skin.

____ ____ ____ _____

     (2) Hold pouch by barrier, center over stoma, and press down gently on barrier. For ambulatory clients, the bottom of the pouch should point toward the client's knees.

____ ____ ____ _____

     (3) Maintain gentle finger pressure around barrier and pouch for 1 to 2 minutes.

____ ____ ____ _____

   b. For two-piece system:
     (1) Apply barrier-paste flange as in steps for one-piece system. Then snap on pouch and maintain finger pressure.

____ ____ ____ _____

10. For both pouching systems, gently tug on the pouch in a downward direction.

____ ____ ____ _____

11. Apply nonallergenic paper tape around skin barrier in a "picture frame" method. Half of the tape should be on the skin barrier and half on the client's skin. Some clients may prefer a belt attached to the pouch.

____ ____ ____ _____

12. Make sure that clients who use ostomy belts can position two fingers between belt and skin.

13. Ostomy deodorant may be added to the pouch.

____ ____ ____ _____

Nurse Alert: Aspirin should never be added to the ostomy pouch as it can cause stomal bleeding.

14. Fold bottom of drainable open-ended pouches up oncc and close using a closure device.

   _____ _____ _____ _____

15. Properly dispose of old pouch and soiled equipment. Remove and discard gloves and wash hands. Consider using room deodorant if needed.

   _____ _____ _____ _____

16. Change pouch every 3 to 7 days unless leaking; pouch can remain in place for tub bath or shower; after bath, pat adhesive dry.

   _____ _____ _____ _____

17. Use Completion Protocol.

   _____ _____ _____ _____

Evaluation

1. Ask client to rate level of comfort around stoma.

   _____ _____ _____ _____

2. Monitor status of stoma.

   _____ _____ _____ _____

3. Auscultate bowel sounds and observe amount, color, consistency, and frequency of fecal elimination from the stoma.

   _____ _____ _____ _____

4. Observe peristomal skin and incision.

   _____ _____ _____ _____

5. Observe integrity of skin barrier and pouching system. Check bag for leakage. Check for seepage around skin barrier.

   _____ _____ _____ _____

6. Observe client's performance of and response to ostomy care.

   _____ _____ _____ _____

• Identify unexpected outcomes and intervene as necessary.

   _____ _____ _____ _____

• Record and report intervention and client's response.

   _____ _____ _____ _____

Performance Checklist: Skill 34.3

Irrigating a Colostomy

	S	U	NP	Comments

Assessment

1. Assess frequency of defecation, character of stool, placement of stoma, and client's regular nutritional pattern.

2. Assess time when client normally irrigates colostomy. With a new ostomy, confer with physician about whether and when irrigations can begin. Obtain written order.

3. Confer with client for best time to irrigate.

4. Assess client's understanding of procedure and ability to perform techniques.

Implementation

1. Use Standard Protocol.

2. Summarize for client how procedure will be performed. Encourage questions as you proceed.

3. Apply gloves. Position client either:
   a. On toilet or in chair in front of toilet, if ambulatory.
   b. On side, with head slightly elevated, if unable to be out of bed.

4. For adult clients, fill irrigation bag with 500 to 1000 ml warm irrigation solution (tap water or saline solution); clear tubing of air by opening flow control clamp and allow solution to run through tubing. Close clamp.

Nurse Alert: Do not use tap water for irrigations if not suitable for drinking. Replace with bottled water.

5. Hang the irrigation solution container on a hook so that the end of the bag is no higher than client's shoulder when sitting or 18 to 20 inches (45-50 cm) above stoma.

6. Remove client's pouch by gently pushing skin from adhesive and barrier; dispose of according to hospital policy for standard

		S	U	NP	Comments

precautions (save clamp if attached to pouch).

7. Place irrigation sleeve over client's stoma. Angle sleeve for appropriate flow of fecal returns. Angle of irrigation sleeve facilitates flow of fecal returns. Adjust belt if used.

8. Lubricate tip of irrigating cone. Reach through the top of the irrigation sleeve and insert the cone gently into the stoma.

Nurse Alert: Only use a cone tip for irrigations. Insert cone securely into stoma to create a seal.

9. With client holding cone, have client open flow control clamp and allow solution to flow. Start with 500 ml; this should take 5 to 10 minutes. Adjust direction of cone to facilitate inflow of solution as needed.

10. If cramping occurs, reduce or stop flow of irrigation fluid.

11. When all the irrigation fluid has been instilled into client's stoma, close flow control clamp and wait 15 seconds before removing irrigation cone from stoma. Close top of irritation sleeve using appropriate closure method. Discard gloves.

12. Allow 15 to 20 minutes for initial evacuation of stool. Keep end of sleeve in toilet or bedpan.

13. Apply gloves. After initial evacuation of stool is over, dry tip of irrigation sleeve and close end with the clip or closure device. Leave in place 30 to 45 minutes while waiting for the secondary evacuation. Client may get off toilet and walk around at this time. Discard gloves.

14. Unclamp sleeve and empty any fecal contents into toilet or bedpan. Rinse sleeve by pouring a small amount of water through the top, then remove sleeve. Rinse with liquid cleanser and cool water. Hang sleeve to dry.

15. Wipe stoma with toilet tissue to remove any stool. Put an appropriate colostomy pouch over stoma. If client is using a two-piece pouching system, place a new flange cap or closed-end pouch onto skin barrier.

16. Use Completion Protocol.

	S	U	NP	Comments

Evaluation

1. Observe the amount and characteristics of the fecal material after irrigation.   ___ ___ ___ _____

2. Evaluate regularity of bowel elimination pattern.   ___ ___ ___ _____

3. Observe client's comfort level and responses.   ___ ___ ___ _____

4. Evaluate client's knowledge of, ability to perform, and response to the irrigation.   ___ ___ ___ _____

- Identify unexpected outcomes and intervene as necessary.   ___ ___ ___ _____

- Record and report intervention and client's response.   ___ ___ ___ _____

Performance Checklist: Skill 35.1

Urinary Catheterization with Indwelling (Retention) Catheter: Female and Male

	S	U	NP	Comments

Assessment

1. Assess client's knowledge and prior experience with catheterization. ____ ____ ____ _____

2. Assess client's weight, age, level of consciousness, ability to cooperate, and mobility of lower extremities. ____ ____ ____ _____

3. Ask client the time of last voiding and to describe urine (if nurse did not observe). Check I&O flow sheet. ____ ____ ____ _____

4. Palpate for bladder over symphysis pubis. ____ ____ ____ _____

5. Inspect perineal region, observing for perineal landmarks, erythema, drainage, or discharge. ____ ____ ____ _____

6. Ask client and check chart for allergies. ____ ____ ____ _____

7. Assess any pathological condition that may impair passage of catheter. ____ ____ ____ _____

8. Review client's medical record, including physician's order and nurse's notes. Note previous catheterization, including catheter size, response of client, and time of last catheterization. ____ ____ ____ _____

Implementation

1. Use Standard Protocol. ____ ____ ____ _____

2. Tell the client you will explain the procedure as you go along. ____ ____ ____ _____

3. Arrange for extra nursing personnel to assist with positioning.
   a. Position female: Dorsal recumbent, draped with bath blanket so only perineum is exposed (alternate: side-lying). ____ ____ ____ _____
   b. Position male: Supine with legs extended, upper body and legs draped with bath blanket or sheet. ____ ____ ____ _____

4. Apply gloves. Cleanse perineal area with soap and water, rinse and dry. ____ ____ ____ _____

	S	U	NP	Comments

5. Position light to illuminate perineum or have assistant hold flashlight.

6. Place catheter kit on overbed table and open outer wrap using sterile technique. If packaged separately, open package containing drainage system; place bag over edge of bottom bed frame and bring tube up between side rail.

7. Put on sterile gloves.

8. Drape the perineum.
   a. With a cuff over both hands, ask client to lift hips and slip drape between client's thighs under buttocks.
   b. Place a second sterile drape with center opening so that perineum is covered and only the genital area is exposed.

9. Arrange supplies on sterile field, maintaining sterility of gloves.
   a. Place closed system outer container with drainage bag, catheter, and attached syringe toward the foot of the bed. If using a closed system, secure bag clamp at this time.
   b. Place top tray with cotton balls, lubricant, and forceps on sterile drape between client's legs.

10. Remove catheter and inject saline into balloon port to check for inflation and leakage.

11. Lubricate catheter 2.5 to 5 cm (1-2 inches) for female and 12.5 to 17.5 cm (5-7 inches) for male.

12. Pour antiseptic solution over all but one cotton ball.

13. Cleanse the urinary meatus with antiseptic solution, holding the cotton ball with the forceps and making a single stroke with each cotton ball.
   a. Female: Separate labia with fingers on nondominant hand (now contaminated). This hand remains in this position for remainder of the procedure. Cleanse labia and meatus using forceps to hold cotton balls and one cotton ball for each stroke, moving anterior to posterior. The first stroke is on one side of meatus, down the center, then on opposite side.

b. Male: Hold shaft of penis at right angle to body with nondominant hand, while retracting foreskin (if present). The nondominant hand, now contaminated, remains in position for the remainder of the procedure. Using forceps to hold cotton ball, cleanse with circular strokes from meatus outward and downward. ____ ____ ____ _____

14. Hold catheter 7.5 to 10 cm (3-4 inches) from tip with dominant hand and slowly insert catheter until urine flows; then advance another 1 to 2 inches. Insert the catheter 5 to 7.5 cm (2-3 inches) for a female and 15 to 17.5 cm (6-7 inches) for a male, while applying traction to penis. Slight resistance may be felt at the prostatic sphincter in the male client. When resistance is met, hold the catheter firmly against the sphincter, without forcing, and catheter should be able to be advanced after a few seconds. ____ ____ ____ _____

15. Hold catheter in place with nondominant hand, use prefilled syringe to inflate balloon. ____ ____ ____ _____

16. Secure indwelling catheter with hypoallergenic tape or catheter strap.
    a. Female: Secure catheter to inner thigh with nonallergenic tape or catheter strap, allowing some slack to prevent tension.
    b. Male: Secure to top of thigh or lower abdomen with tape or catheter strap. Replace foreskin, if present. Note: Connect catheter to drainage bag if not previously connected. ____ ____ ____ _____

17. Position drainage bag lower than bladder with tubing coiled on the bed (not in dependent loops). ____ ____ ____ _____

18. Cleanse and dry perineal area. Position client for comfort. ____ ____ ____ _____

19. Measure urine, noting color and clarity. ____ ____ ____ _____

Nurse Alert: Agency policy may restrict maximum volume of urine to be drained at one time to 800 to 1000 ml. Rapid emptying of an extremely distended bladder can result in shock.

20. Use Completion Protocol. ____ ____ ____ _____

Evaluation

1. Palpate bladder and observe urine in catheter bag for amount, color, and clarity. ____ ____ ____ _____

	S	U	NP	Comments

2. Determine client's comfort level. _____ _____ _____ _____

3. Measure I&O. _____ _____ _____ _____

- Identify unexpected outcomes and
  intervene as necessary. _____ _____ _____ _____

- Record and report intervention and
  client's response. _____ _____ _____ _____

Name _____   Date _____   Instructor's Name _____

Performance Checklist: Procedural Guideline 35-1

Removal of an Indwelling Catheter

	S	U	NP	Comments

Assessment

1. Check physician's order. _____ _____ _____ _____

2. Note length of time catheter was in place. _____ _____ _____ _____

3. Assess client's knowledge of what to expect. _____ _____ _____ _____

Implementation

1. Use Standard Protocol. _____ _____ _____ _____

2. Apply gloves. Position client supine and place a waterproof pad under the catheter. Females will need to abduct the legs with the drape between the thighs. Drape can lie over male client's legs. _____ _____ _____ _____

3. Insert hub of syringe into inflation valve (balloon port). Aspirate until tubing collapses, indicating that entire contents of balloon have been removed. _____ _____ _____ _____

4. Remove catheter steadily and smoothly. _____ _____ _____ _____

Nurse Alert: Catheter should slide out very easily. Do not pull. If resistance is felt, repeat step 3 to remove remaining fluid in balloon.

5. Wrap catheter in waterproof pad. Unhook collection bag and drainage tubing from bed. _____ _____ _____ _____

6. Measure urine and empty the drainage bag. Record output. _____ _____ _____ _____

7. Cleanse the perineum with soap and water and dry thoroughly. _____ _____ _____ _____

8. Place the urine "hat" on the toilet seat. _____ _____ _____ _____

9. Use Completion Protocol. _____ _____ _____ _____

Evaluation

1. Observe time and amount of first voided specimen. _____ _____ _____ _____

2. Monitor I&O. _____ _____ _____ _____

3. Ask client to list the signs and symptoms of urinary tract infection. _____ _____ _____ _____

	S	U	NP	Comments

- Identify unexpected outcomes and intervene as necessary.   _____ _____ _____ _____

- Record and report intervention and client's response.   _____ _____ _____ _____

408

Performance Checklist: Skill 35.2

Inserting Straight Catheter for Specimen Collection or Residual

	S	U	NP	Comments

Assessment

1. Review intake and output record.

2. Ask client to describe any discomfort experienced while voiding.

3. Review physician's orders.

4. Identify time client voids.

5. Assess client's knowledge and experience with urinary retention and catheterization.

Implementation

1. Use Standard Protocol.

2. Ask client to void completely and measure volume of urine.

3. Immediately after voiding, position and drape client as for insertion of an indwelling catheter.

4. While standing on the appropriate side of the bed (depending on whether right- or left-handed), open catheterization kit using sterile technique, and place outer plastic bag within reach.

5. Apply sterile gloves.

6. Organize sterile supplies and pour antiseptic solution into compartment containing sterile cotton balls.

7. Open lubricant packet and lubricate tip of catheter.

8. Apply sterile drape, keeping gloves sterile.

9. Using sterile technique, place sterile tray and contents on sterile drape between client's legs.

10. Open specimen container, if needed, and place within easy reach of distal end of catheter.

11. Cleanse urethral meatus.

409

Nurse Alert: Carefully inspect the perineum and visualize the urinary meatus.

12. Pick up catheter with gloved dominant hand 2 to 3 inches from catheter tip. Hold catheter loosely coiled in palm of hand.   _____ _____ _____ _____

13. Insert catheter until urine flows.   _____ _____ _____ _____

14. Collect 10 to 30 ml of urine in specimen container, then allow remaining urine to collect in outer container of package.   _____ _____ _____ _____

15. Allow bladder to empty fully unless agency policy restricts maximum volume of urine to be drained.   _____ _____ _____ _____

16. Steadily and smoothly remove straight catheter.   _____ _____ _____ _____

17. Assist client to a comfortable position. Wash and dry perineal area.   _____ _____ _____ _____

18. Accurately measure urine that is obtained.   _____ _____ _____ _____

19. Use Completion Protocol.   _____ _____ _____ _____

Evaluation

1. Observe amount of urine obtained.   _____ _____ _____ _____

2. Observe characteristics of urine specimen.   _____ _____ _____ _____

3. Ask client to describe level of comfort.   _____ _____ _____ _____

4. Ask client to describe the purpose of the procedure.   _____ _____ _____ _____

• Identify unexpected outcomes and intervene as necessary.   _____ _____ _____ _____

• Record and report intervention and client's response.   _____ _____ _____ _____

Performance Checklist: Skill 35.3

Continuous Bladder Irrigation

	S	U	NP	Comments

Assessment

1. Assess client's level of consciousness and ability to cooperate.

2. Palpate bladder for distention and tenderness.

3. Ask client about the presence of bladder pain or spasms.

4. Observe the characteristics of the urine.

5. Review intake and output (I&O) record.

6. Assess client's knowledge about catheter irrigation.

Implementation

1. Use Standard Protocol.

2. Place label or irrigation solution bag with client's name, room number, date, and time. Mark bag FOR GU IRRIGATION ONLY in red, type of solution, and any additives.

3. Hang bag on IV pole.

4. Insert tip (spike) of sterile irrigation tubing into bag containing irrigation solution.

5. Close clamp on tubing and fill the drip chamber one-half full by squeezing the chamber. Open the clamp to completely fill tubing and remove air. Close the clamp.

6. Apply gloves. Wipe off irrigation port of triple-lumen catheter with antiseptic swab and connect to irrigation tubing aseptically.

Nurse Alert: Be sure drainage tubing is patent.

7. Calculate drip rate and adjust rate at roller clamp (according to physician's orders or agency protocol).

8. If urine is bright red or has clots, increase irrigation rate until drainage appears pink.

9. Replace bag of irrigation solution as needed.

	S	U	NP	Comments
10. Using gloves, empty catheter bag as needed.	___	___	___	_____
11. Compare urine output with irrigation solution's infusion every hour.	___	___	___	_____
12. Use Completion Protocol.	___	___	___	_____

Evaluation

	S	U	NP	Comments
1. Measure urine output by subtracting total irrigation solution from total drainage in bag.	___	___	___	_____
2. Evaluate the characteristics and amount of urine output.	___	___	___	_____
3. Ask if client is experiencing pain and assess for signs and symptoms of an infection.	___	___	___	_____
• Identify unexpected outcomes and intervene as necessary.	___	___	___	_____
• Record and report intervention and client's response.	___	___	___	_____

Performance Checklist: Skill 35.4

Suprapubic Catheters

	S	U	NP	Comments

Assessment

1. Assess catheter insertion site for erythema, edema, drainage, and odor.

2. Assess characteristics and amount of urine (color, clarity, odor).

3. Assess for fever and chills.

4. Assess tape site for irritation.

5. Identify allergies.

6. Assess client's level of comfort.

Implementation

1. Use Standard Protocol.

2. Apply gloves. Remove old dressing and place dressing and gloves in bag.

3. Put on sterile gloves.

4. Assess insertion site and patency of catheter.

5. Without creating tension, hold catheter erect with nondominant hand while cleansing site in a circular motion, starting closest to the catheter site and continuing in outward widening circles for approximately 2 inches (5 cm).

6. Take one fresh gauze pad moistened in antiseptic solution and cleanse base of catheter, working from proximal to distal.

7. With sterile gloved hand, apply split gauze around catheter and tape in place.

8. Secure catheter to abdomen with tape or Velcro multipurpose tube holder to reduce tension on insertion site.

9. Coil excess tubing on bed and secure to dressing. Keep drainage bag below level of the bladder. Ensure bag and catheter junctions are securely in place.

	S	U	NP	Comments

10. Suprapubic catheter may be clamped for several hours per physician's order. _____ _____ _____ _____

11. Unclamp catheter if client is unable to void and feels full. Re-clamp per physician's order. _____ _____ _____ _____

12. Evaluate amount of residual urine after client has voided normally with catheter clamped. _____ _____ _____ _____

13. Use Completion Protocol. _____ _____ _____ _____

Evaluation

1. Monitor suprapubic catheter output. _____ _____ _____ _____

2. Monitor for signs of infection (fever, elevated white blood cell count). _____ _____ _____ _____

3. Inspect insertion site and surrounding skin. _____ _____ _____ _____

4. Determine client's comfort level. _____ _____ _____ _____

5. Observe client's ability to care for insertion site and drainage bag. _____ _____ _____ _____

6. Ask client to state signs and symptoms of a urinary tract and insertion site infection. _____ _____ _____ _____

• Identify unexpected outcomes and intervene as necessary. _____ _____ _____ _____

• Record and report intervention and client's response. _____ _____ _____ _____

Performance Checklist: Skill 35.5

Urinary Diversions (Continent and Incontinent)

	S	U	NP	Comments

Assessment

1. Inspect pouch for amount of urine, leakage, and length of time in place.

2. Observe stoma site for color, moistness, or irritation, and check peristomal skin for maceration. Inspect all external suture lines for healing progress.

3. Observe and palpate skin around stoma for erythema, excoriation, edema, and drainage.

4. Assess level of comfort of client.

5. Observe abdominal contours, folds, and suture line.

6. Assess client's emotional response and knowledge of ostomy care.

Implementation

1. Use Standard Protocol.

2. Position client supine to allow for easy access to stoma so that abdomen is as smooth or flat as possible. Be sure client can view procedure.

3. Prepare pouch by removing backing from barrier and adhesive. Cut opening $1/16$ to $1/8$ inch larger than stoma before removing backing.

4. Apply gloves. Place a towel or disposable waterproof barrier under client. Tightly roll several gauze pads separately to form "wicks."

5. Remove used pouch gently by pushing skin away from barrier, avoiding any tension on stents (if present). Immediately place a gauze wick over stoma. Place sterile gauze pad underneath tips of stents, if present.

Nurse Alert: Avoid tension on stents, if present.

6. Cleanse skin around the stoma gently with warm tap water using gauze pads. Do not scrub skin. Wick stoma continuously.

    ___ ___ ___ _____

7. Saturate a washcloth with a solution of $\frac{1}{3}$ vinegar and $\frac{2}{3}$ warm water if uric acid crystals are present. Soak the involved area for several minutes. Rinse with warm tap water and dry completely with dry gauze or towel. Remove any mucus from stoma.

    ___ ___ ___ _____

8. Use barrier paste or seal to fill in creases that have formed next to stoma. Allow to dry 1 to 2 minutes.

    ___ ___ ___ _____

9. Apply skin sealant in circular area around base of stoma to skin not protected by barrier and let dry.

    ___ ___ ___ _____

10. Hold pouch by barrier, center over stoma and stents, and press down gently. Bottom of pouch is angled slightly to attach to bedside urinary drainage bag.

    ___ ___ ___ _____

11. Use another skin sealant on skin in contact with adhesive and allow to dry. Press adhesive backing smoothly against skin, starting from the bottom and working up and around the sides.

    ___ ___ ___ _____

12. Maintain gentle finger pressure around barrier for 1 to 2 minutes.

    ___ ___ ___ _____

13. If using a two-piece pouch, apply flange as above, then snap on pouch. If client is mostly ambulatory, apply pouch vertically.

    ___ ___ ___ _____

14. Dispose of used pouch and soiled equipment in a plastic bag and place it in appropriate receptacle.

    ___ ___ ___ _____

15. Empty bag when $\frac{1}{2}$ to $\frac{2}{3}$ full of urine. Measure and record urine output. Secure clamp on end of bag opening for repeated emptying.

    ___ ___ ___ _____

16. Use Completion Protocol.

    ___ ___ ___ _____

Evaluation

1. Evaluate amount and characteristics of urine.

    ___ ___ ___ _____

2. Inspect and palpate condition of stoma (color, edema, tenderness).

    ___ ___ ___ _____

3. Observe peristomal skin (excoriation, erythema).

    ___ ___ ___ _____

4. Ask client to rate level of comfort.

    ___ ___ ___ _____

	S	U	NP	Comments

5. Ask client to view stoma and observe ability to perform pouch care at next change.

    ____ ____ ____ _____

• Identify unexpected outcomes and intervene as necessary.

    ____ ____ ____ _____

• Record and report intervention and client's response.

    ____ ____ ____ _____

Performance Checklist: Skill 36.1

Caring for an Eye Prosthesis

	S	U	NP	Comments

Assessment

1. Determine which eye is artificial (no reaction to light). ____ ____ ____ _____

2. Inspect surrounding tissues of eyelid and eye socket for inflammation, tenderness, swelling, or drainage after prosthesis removal. Wear gloves if drainage is suspected or present. ____ ____ ____ _____

3. Assess client's routines for prosthetic care: frequency and methods of cleaning. ____ ____ ____ _____

4. Assess client's ability to remove, clean, and reinsert prosthesis. ____ ____ ____ _____

Implementation

1. Use Standard Protocol. ____ ____ ____ _____

2. Apply gloves. With thumb, gently retract lower eyelid against orbital ridge. ____ ____ ____ _____

3. Exert slight pressure below eyelid. If prosthesis does not slide out, use bulb syringe or medicine dropper bulb to apply direct suction to prosthesis. ____ ____ ____ _____

4. Place prosthesis in palm of hand and clean with mild soap and water or plain saline by rubbing between thumb and index finger. ____ ____ ____ _____

5. Rinse well under running tap water and dry with soft washcloth or facial tissue. ____ ____ ____ _____

6. If client is not to have prosthesis reinserted, store in sterile saline or water in plastic storage case. Label with client's name and room number. ____ ____ ____ _____

7. Clean eyelid margins and socket.

   a. Retract upper and lower eyelids with thumb and index finger. (Inspection can be done at this time.) ____ ____ ____ _____

   b. Wash socket with washcloth or gauze square moistened in warm water or saline. ____ ____ ____ _____

	S	U	NP	Comments

c. Dry socket well with gauze pads.

d. Wash eyelids with mild soap and water, wiping from inner to outer canthus, using a clean part of cloth with each wipe. Dry eyelids using the same method.

Nurse Alert: Place moistened cloth over eyelids for several minutes during cleaning to remove crusts.

8. Moisten prosthesis with water or saline.

9. Retract client's upper eyelid with index finger or thumb of nondominant hand.

10. With dominant hand, hold prosthesis so that notched or pointed edge is positioned toward nose. Iris faces outward.

11. Slide prosthesis up under upper eyelid as far as possible. Then push down lower lid to allow prosthesis to slip into place.

Nurse Alert: Do not force prosthesis into socket.

12. Gently wipe away excess fluid if necessary.

13. Use Completion Protocol.

Evaluation

1. Determine client's feelings about prosthesis and ability to perform care.

2. Inspect eyelids and eye socket for integrity.

3. Inspect for any signs of infection.

4. Ask client about comfort level.

5. Observe client performing self-care for prosthesis.

• Identify unexpected outcomes and intervene as necessary.

• Record and report intervention and client's response.

Name _____ Date _____ Instructor's Name _____

Performance Checklist: Skill 36.2

Eye Irrigations

	S	U	NP	Comments

Assessment

1. Assess reason for eye irrigation. _____ _____ _____ _____

2. Assess the eye for redness, excessive tearing, and discharge. Assess the eyelids and lacrimal glands for edema. Ask client about itching, burning, pain, blurred vision, or photophobia. _____ _____ _____ _____

3. Assess client's ability to cooperate. Extra assistance may be needed. _____ _____ _____ _____

Implementation

1. Use Standard Protocol. _____ _____ _____ _____

2. Apply gloves. Reassure client that eye can be closed periodically and that no object will touch eye. Remove contact lenses if possible. _____ _____ _____ _____

3. Assist client to side-lying position on the same side as the affected eye. Turn head toward affected eye. _____ _____ _____ _____

4. Place waterproof pad under client's face. _____ _____ _____ _____

5. With cotton ball moistened in prescribed solution (or normal saline), gently clean eyelid margins and eyelashes from inner to outer canthus. _____ _____ _____ _____

6. Place curved emesis basin just below client's cheek on the side of affected eye. _____ _____ _____ _____

7. With gloved finger gently retract upper and lower eyelids to expose the conjunctival sacs. To hold lids open, apply pressure to lower bony orbit and bony prominence beneath eyebrow. Do not apply pressure over eye. _____ _____ _____ _____

8. Hold irrigating syringe, dropper, or IV tubing approximately 1 inch (2.5 cm) from the inner canthus. _____ _____ _____ _____

9. Ask client to look up. Gently irrigate with a steady stream toward the lower conjunctival sac to the outer canthus. _____ _____ _____ _____

	S	U	NP	Comments

10. Allow client to close the eye periodically. ____ ____ ____ _____

11. Continue irrigation until all solution is used or secretions have been cleared. (NOTE: A 15-minute irrigation is needed to flush chemicals.) ____ ____ ____ _____

12. Dry eyelids and facial area with sterile cotton ball. ____ ____ ____ _____

13. Use Completion Protocol. ____ ____ ____ _____

Evaluation

1. Evaluate client's comfort level and visual perception. ____ ____ ____ _____

2. Evaluate level of anxiety. ____ ____ ____ _____

3. Ask if vision is blurred after irrigation. ____ ____ ____ _____

4. Observe pupillary reaction and extraocular movement. ____ ____ ____ _____

• Identify unexpected outcomes and intervene as necessary. ____ ____ ____ _____

• Record and report intervention and client's response. ____ ____ ____ _____

Performance Checklist: Skill 36.3

Caring for Clients with Hearing Aids

	S	U	NP	Comments

Assessment

1. Assess client's knowledge of and routines for cleansing and caring for hearing aid. ____ ____ ____ _____

2. Observe whether client can hear clearly with use of aid by talking slowly and clearly in normal tone of voice. ____ ____ ____ _____

3. Assess if hearing aid is working by removing from client's ear. Close battery case and turn volume slowly to high. Cup hand over hearing aid. If squealing sound (feedback) is heard, it is working. If no sound is heard, replace batteries and test again. ____ ____ ____ _____

4. Inspect ear mold for cracked or rough edges. ____ ____ ____ _____

5. Inspect for accumulation of cerumen around aid and plugging of opening in aid. ____ ____ ____ _____

Implementation

1. Use Standard Protocol. ____ ____ ____ _____

2. Have equipment at bedside for client to see. ____ ____ ____ _____

3. Cleaning hearing aid:

   a. Wipe aid with soft washcloth. Use wax loop or brush (supplied with aid) or tip of syringe needle to clean the holes in the aid; do not jam wax deeper into holes. ____ ____ ____ _____

Nurse Alert: Protect device from moisture, heat, breakage, and loss.

   b. Open battery door and allow it to air dry. ____ ____ ____ _____
   c. Wash ear canal with washcloth moistened in soap and water. Rinse and dry. ____ ____ ____ _____
   d. If hearing aid is to be stored, place in dry storage case with desiccant material. Label case with client's name and room number. If more than one aid, note right or left. Turn off hearing aid when not in use. ____ ____ ____ _____

	S	U	NP	Comments

4. Inserting hearing aid:
   a. Check batteries.
   b. Turn aid off and volume control down.
   c. Hold aid so that the long portion with the hole(s) is at the bottom.
   d. Insert bore into the canal first. Use other hand to pull up and back on outer ear. Gently twist and push aid into ear until it is in place and fits snugly in the midline. Ask client if comfortably placed.
   e. Adjust volume gradually to comfortable level for talking to client in regular voice 3 to 4 feet away. Rotate volume control toward nose to increase volume and away from nose to decrease volume. Note that some ITC hearing aids have preset sound levels that require a special instrument to adjust. Most clients leave setting at an acceptable level.

Nurse Alert: Programmable aids have volume control located on the remote. For most clients, aids work best at lower volume settings.

5. Use Completion Protocol.

Evaluation

1. Observe client's response to conversational tone.

2. Observe response to environmental sounds.

3. Observe client's ability to perform hearing aid care.

4. Ask about comfort after hearing aid insertion.

• Identify unexpected outcomes and intervene as necessary.

• Record and report intervention and client's response.

Performance Checklist: Skill 36.4

Ear Irrigations

	S	U	NP	Comments

Assessment

1. Review prescriber's order for solution and ear to be irrigated. ___ ___ ___ _____

2. Review medical history for ruptured tympanic membrane, myringotomy tubes, or surgery of auditory canal. ___ ___ ___ _____

3. Inspect the pinna and external auditory meatus for redness, swelling, drainage, abrasions, and presence of cerumen or foreign objects. ___ ___ ___ _____

4. Use an otoscope to inspect deeper portions of the auditory canal. ___ ___ ___ _____

5. Assess client's comfort level. ___ ___ ___ _____

6. Assess client's hearing ability in the affected ear. ___ ___ ___ _____

7. Assess client's knowledge of proper ear care. ___ ___ ___ _____

Implementation

1. Use Standard Protocol. ___ ___ ___ _____

2. Apply gloves. Assist client to a sitting or lying position with head turned toward the affected ear. Place towel or waterproof pad under client's head and shoulder. Have client help hold basin under affected ear. ___ ___ ___ _____

3. Pour prescribed irrigating solution into sterile basin. Check the temperature of the solution (98.6° F or 37° C) by pouring a small drop on your inner forearm. ___ ___ ___ _____

4. Gently clean auricle and outer ear canal with moistened cotton applicator. Do not force drainage or cerumen into ear canal. ___ ___ ___ _____

Nurse Alert: Tell client not to make sudden moves.

5. Fill syringe and expel air. If using dental irrigating device, use low setting. ___ ___ ___ _____

6. With nondominant hand, straighten the auditory meatus by gently drawing the

pinna up and back (for adult) or down and back (for young child). Place the tip of the irrigating device just inside the external meatus. Leave a space around the irrigating tip and canal.

7. Direct the fluid gently toward the posterior wall of the ear canal.

8. Maintain the flow of the irrigation in a steady stream until you see small two large pieces of cerumen flow from the canal.

9. Periodically ask if the client is experiencing pain, nausea, or vertigo.

10. Drain excessive fluid from the ear by having client tilt the head toward the affected side.

11. Dry the canal gently with a cotton-tipped applicator and then chemically dry with an antiseptic otic solution. Remove and discard gloves and wash hands.

12. Use Completion Protocol.

Evaluation

1. Monitor pain level during irrigation.

2. Monitor pain level after irrigation.

3. Observe for verbal and nonverbal signs of anxiety during the procedure.

4. Inspect external meatus and ear canal.

5. Assess hearing acuity after irrigation.

• Identify unexpected outcomes and intervene as necessary.

• Record and report intervention and client's response.

Performance Checklist: Skill 37.1

Resuscitation

	S	U	NP	Comments

Assessment

1. Assess the client's unresponsiveness by shaking the client and shouting, "Are you OK?" ____ ____ ____ _____

2. Activate the emergency medical services according to agency policy and procedure. ____ ____ ____ _____

Implementation

1. Assess responsiveness and call for help. ____ ____ ____ _____

2. Observe for signs of circulation and chest movement; listen and feel for breaths. ____ ____ ____ _____

Nurse Alert: Be aware if client has Do Not Resuscitate order.

3. Open the airway.
   a. If no head or neck trauma is suspected, use the head-tilt, chin-lift method. ____ ____ ____ _____
   b. If head or neck trauma is suspected, use the jaw-thrust maneuver only. Grasp angles of client's lower jaw and lift with both hands, displacing the mandible forward. ____ ____ ____ _____

4. If client is breathing and no trauma is present, place client in the recovery position. ____ ____ ____ _____

5. If no respirations are detected, call for assistance. ____ ____ ____ _____

6. Apply gloves. Place victim supine on hard surface, such as floor or ground, or use the backboard found on the resuscitation cart or the headboard of the hospital bed. If the client must be moved to the supine position, use the log-rolling technique to maintain spinal integrity. ____ ____ ____ _____

7. Correctly position for resuscitative efforts.
   a. One-person rescue: Face client while kneeling parallel to the client's sternum. ____ ____ ____ _____
   b. Two-person rescue: One person faces client while kneeling parallel to the client's head. Second person is on the

	S	U	NP	Comments

opposite side parallel to the client's sternum.

8. Mouth-to-mouth artificial respirations
   a. *Adult*
      (1) Pinch client's nose with thumb and index finger and occlude mouth with rescuer's mouth, face shield, or CPR pocket mask. Attempt two slow breaths, 1½ to 2 seconds per breath.
      (2) The rescuer should take a breath after each ventilation.
      (3) Allow the client to exhale between breaths.
      (4) Continue with 12 breaths per minute.
   b. *Child* (1-8 years of age)
      (1) Pinch the victim's nose tightly with thumb and forefinger. Place rescuer's mouth, face shield, or CPR pocket mask over client's mouth, forming an airtight seal. Give two slow breaths, 1 to 1½ seconds per breath.
      (2) Pause after the first breath to take a breath.
      (3) Continue with 20 breaths per minute.
   c. *Infant*
      (1) Place the rescuer's mouth, face shield, or CPR pocket mask over the infant's nose and mouth, forming an airtight seal.
      (2) Give two breaths slowly at 1 to 1½ seconds per breath.
      (3) Continue with 20 breaths per minute.

9. Bag-valve-mask artificial respirations
   a. *All ages*
      (1) Connect oxygen supply tubing to bag-valve-mask and oxygen flow meter. Adjust oxygen to 100% F_IO_2 or ordered rate.
      (2) Insert oropharyngeal airway, if available.
      (3) Position the face mask of the bag-valve-mask over the client's mouth and nose.
      (4) Give slow breaths by squeezing the bag. Observe for chest movement.
      (5) Allow time for client to exhale.

10. If ventilation attempt is unsuccessful, reposition the client's head and reattempt rescue breathing again. If ventilation attempt remains unsuccessful, the airway may be obstructed by a foreign body that will need to be removed.

    a. *Adult:* Begin with 5 abdominal thrusts below xiphoid and above navel. Open victim's mouth by grasping both the tongue and lower jaw between the thumb and fingers and lifting. Finger sweep: Using index finger of opposite hand, sweep back of mouth and throat. Maneuver object into mouth for removal. If this is unsuccessful, give 2 breaths, reposition head, give 2 more breaths, and repeat until airway is cleared.   ____ ____ ____ _____

    b. *Child:* Abdominal thrusts are recommended, without finger sweeps unless the object can be visualized.   ____ ____ ____ _____

    c. *Infant:* Back blows and chest thrusts are recommended. Do not perform blind finger sweeps.   ____ ____ ____ _____

11. Suction secretions as needed or turn client's head to the side if no trauma is suspected.   ____ ____ ____ _____

12. Check for the presence of carotid pulse in adult and child or brachial pulse in infant. Feel for 3 to 5 seconds.   ____ ____ ____ _____

13. If no pulse, initiate chest compressions.   ____ ____ ____ _____

Nurse Alert: Ensure fingers are off the ribs and lowermost part of xiphoid process.

    a. *Adult:* Place heel of hands, one atop the other, on lower third of the sternum. Lock elbows and maintain shoulders in line with sternum.   ____ ____ ____ _____

    b. *Child:* Place the heel of one hand on the lower half of the sternum. Maintain open airway with other hand, if possible.   ____ ____ ____ _____

    c. *Infant:* Place two or three fingers on the lower half of the sternum just below the level of the infant's nipples.   ____ ____ ____ _____

14. Compress chest downward to proper depth and then release. Maintain constant contact with skin.

    a. *Adult:* $1\frac{1}{2}$ to 2 inches (4-5 cm)   ____ ____ ____ _____

    b. *Child:* 1 to $1\frac{1}{2}$ inches (2.5-4 cm)   ____ ____ ____ _____

    c. *Infant:* $\frac{1}{2}$ to 1 inch (1-2.5 cm)   ____ ____ ____ _____

15. Maintain correct ratio proportionate to number of rescuers: One or two rescuers: 15 compressions, 2 breaths.

	S	U	NP	Comments

a. *Adult:* minimum of 80 to 100 compressions per minute

b. *Child:* minimum of 100 compressions per minute

c. *Infant:* minimum of 100 compressions per minute

16. Continue artificial respiration.

17. Monitor the adequacy of the compressions during two-rescuer CPR with palpation of the carotid (adult, child) or brachial (infant) pulse during compressions. Have the rescuer performing the breathing palpate the pulse during compression. Do not delay compression.

18. Continue CPR until the rescuer is relieved, client regains cardiopulmonary function independently, or physician directs that CPR be discontinued.

19. Use Completion Protocol.

Evaluation

1. Inspect chest wall for rise and fall during breathing. Monitor for adequate seal over client's mouth.

2. Palpate for presence of pulse after 4 cycles of compressions and breaths.

3. Observe for return of respiration and circulation.

• Identify unexpected outcomes and intervene as necessary.

• Record and report intervention and client's response.

Name _Hien Dang._   Date _____   Instructor's Name _ABottok,RN._

Performance Checklist: Skill 37.2

Code Management

	S	U	NP	Comments

Assessment

1. Assess client's unresponsiveness. ____ ____ ____ _____

2. Activate the emergency medical service in accordance with hospital policy and procedure. ____ ____ ____ _____

3. Begin CPR efforts. ____ ____ ____ _____

Implementation

1. Follow Skill 37.1. Establish absence of respirations, begin artificial respirations, establish absence of pulse, and begin compressions (ABC). ____ ____ ____ _____

Nurse Alert: Skill requires that you be aware of client's code status, that CPR be performed immediately after discovery of client with an arrest, and that electrical defibrillation equipment be obtained as soon as possible.

2. First available person brings the resuscitation cart with emergency drugs, intubation equipment, IV access supplies, and other equipment. ____ ____ ____ _____

3. Apply gloves. If an automatic external defibrillator (AED) is available, attach to client and deliver shock.
   a. Turn on the power. ____ ____ ____ _____
   b. Attach the device. Stop CPR and attach one pad to the right of the sternum just below the clavicle and the other to the left of the precordium. Ensure that cables are connected to the AED. ____ ____ ____ _____
   c. Initiate analysis of the rhythm. Each brand of AED is different, so familiarity with the model is important. Clear rescuers and bystanders from the victim. ____ ____ ____ _____
   d. Announce to clear the victim and check to see no one is in contact before pressing shock button. Deliver the shock in a series of three as indicated by the AED.

	S	U	NP	Comments

The AED has a pause time of 5 to 15 seconds for rhythm analysis.

e. Check for pulse after three shocks. If no pulse, resume CPR for 1 minute, then begin the shock sequence again.

4. Have someone assist the client's roommate away from the code scene.

5. Have client's chart available. The client's nurse must relay information about the client to the team. This information includes events occurring immediately before the arrest, vital signs, laboratory results, radiology findings, and medications. The code leader may want information about the location of family members.

6. If respirations are absent but pulse is present, assist the code team to:
   a. Administer oxygen at high flow rate by mask or bag-valve-mask.
   b. Monitor vital signs, including cardiac rhythm via resuscitation monitor.
   c. Prepare for endotracheal intubation.
   d. Establish intravenous (IV) access with a large-bore needle and begin infusion of 0.9% normal saline (NS).
   e. Assist ancillary team to obtain blood samples, including arterial blood gases (ABGs).
   f. Review history for suspected causes of cardiac arrest.

7. If respirations and pulse are absent and no AED is available, assist the code team to:
   a. Prepare for defibrillation and defibrillate. Defibrillation is performed only by personnel trained and certified to do so.
   b. Defibrillator is turned on and proper energy level is selected.
   c. Conductive materials (electrode gel or defibrillator gel pads) are applied to client's chest where defibrillator paddles will be placed.
   d. Paddles are charged and placed on the client's chest wall with one to the right of the sternum just below the clavicle and the other to the left of the precordium.
   e. Operator applies a firm pressure to the paddles, announces intent to shock the client, and makes sure no personnel are directly or indirectly in contact with the client.

	S	U	NP	Comments

Nurse Alert: Verify that no one is in contact with the client.

    f. Operator depresses the buttons on the defibrillator paddles at the same time to discharge the electrical current. ____ ____ ____ _____

    g. The first defibrillation activity is performed as a rapidly repeated series of three if the monitor displays persistent ventricular fibrillation or ventricular tachycardia without a pulse. ____ ____ ____ _____

8. If three shocks fail or a different dysrhythmia is present:
    a. Continue CPR.
    b. Establish IV access.
    c. Administer medications.
    d. Establish ventilation (intubation).
    e. Repeat shocks if warranted.

9. If not involved in the performance of CPR, nurse should obtain supplies and drugs as requested.

10. Anticipate the types of vasoactive medications that will likely be used. Double-check dosages to be given.

11. Remain in the room during the resuscitative phase.

12. Keep unnecessary personnel out of the room during the resuscitative phase.

13. Ensure all interventions, medication administration, and client responses are being recorded.

14. Continue resuscitation efforts until client regains pulse or until the physician determines cessation of efforts.

15. Use Completion Protocol.

Evaluation

1. Inspect the client's chest wall for movement during artificial respiration.

2. Observe pulse oximetry levels, if available.

3. Assess pulse during chest compressions to determine adequacy.

4. Observe for possible rib fractures from compressions.

	S	U	NP	Comments
• Identify unexpected outcomes and intervene as necessary.	___	___	___	_____
• Record and report intervention and client's response.	___	___	___	_____

Performance Checklist: Skill 38.1

Managing Central Venous Lines

	S	U	NP	Comments

Assessment

1. Assess client for indications for long-term device. _____ _____ _____ _____

2. Assess baseline for vital signs and I&O. _____ _____ _____ _____

3. Assess catheter patency. _____ _____ _____ _____

4. Assess insertion site for integrity. _____ _____ _____ _____

Implementation

1. Use Standard Protocol. _____ _____ _____ _____

2. Insertion site care
   a. Provide care every 24 to 48 hours and prn for gauze dressings and every 7 days and prn for transparent dressings. _____ _____ _____ _____
   b. Explain procedure to client. _____ _____ _____ _____
   c. Don mask. _____ _____ _____ _____
   d. Apply gloves. Remove old dressing and tape. Discard in receptacle. _____ _____ _____ _____
   e. Inspect the catheter, insertion site, suture, and surrounding skin. _____ _____ _____ _____
   f. Remove and discard nonsterile gloves; apply sterile gloves. _____ _____ _____ _____
   g. Using combination swab, cleanse catheter and site, working outward in a circular motion, or follow steps i and j. _____ _____ _____ _____
   h. Using alcohol swab, cleanse catheter and site, working outward in a circular motion. Repeat 2 times; allow to dry completely. Use chlorhexidine if client is allergic to alcohol. _____ _____ _____ _____
   i. Using povidone-iodine swab, cleanse catheter and site, working outward in a circular motion. Repeat with new swab. Allow to dry completely. Use chlorhexidine if client is allergic to povidone-iodine. _____ _____ _____ _____
   j. Apply sterile gauze or clear occlusive dressing. _____ _____ _____ _____
   k. Tape dressing in "window-frame" fashion as needed. _____ _____ _____ _____

l. For PICC lines, coil extension tubing and tape securely to client's arm.

m. Write the date, time, and your initials on the label.

____ ____ ____ _____

n. Clamp lumens one at a time and remove injection caps.

____ ____ ____ _____

o. Cleanse ports with povidone-iodine and allow to dry completely.

____ ____ ____ _____

p. Put new caps in place. Open clamps for infusion.

____ ____ ____ _____

3. Blood drawing through insertion cap

a. Use Standard Protocol.

____ ____ ____ _____

b. Explain procedure to client.

____ ____ ____ _____

c. Cleanse injection cap with povidone-iodine and allow to dry completely.

____ ____ ____ _____

d. Stop intravenous (IV) infusion.
NOTE: If infusion is critical for client's well-being, draw blood peripherally.

____ ____ ____ _____

e. Flush catheter port with 5 ml NS.

____ ____ ____ _____

f. Aspirate 3 to 5 ml blood and discard or attach vacutainer device and draw a red-top blood tube for discard.

____ ____ ____ _____

g. Aspirate specimen and place in appropriate laboratory tube(s).

____ ____ ____ _____

h. Flush catheter with 10 ml saline solution.

____ ____ ____ _____

i. Flush catheter port with 3 ml heparin solution.

____ ____ ____ _____

j. Clamp lumen and remove cap.

____ ____ ____ _____

k. Cleanse port with povidone-iodine and allow to dry completely.

____ ____ ____ _____

4. Removal of central venous catheter

a. Use Standard Protocol.

____ ____ ____ _____

b. Explain procedure to client.

____ ____ ____ _____

c. Place client in supine or Trendelenburg position.

____ ____ ____ _____

d. Place moisture-proof underpad beneath site.

____ ____ ____ _____

e. Apply gloves. Remove old dressing and tape

____ ____ ____ _____

f. Clean site using povidone-iodine swabs, starting at site and working outward in a circular motion. Allow to air dry.

____ ____ ____ _____

g. If sutures are present, open suture removal set.

____ ____ ____ _____

h. With nondominant hand, grasp suture with forceps. Using dominant hand, cut suture carefully with sterile scissors, making sure to avoid damage to skin or catheter. Lift suture out and discard.

____ ____ ____ _____

i. Using nondominant hand, apply sterile 4×4 gauze to site. Instruct client to take deep breath as catheter is withdrawn.

     ____ ____ ____   _____

j. With dominant hand, remove catheter in a smooth, continuous motion. Apply pressure to site immediately and continue for 5 to 10 minutes. Observe for bleeding.

     ____ ____ ____   _____

k. Apply sterile dressing to site. Write the date, time, and initials on dressing.

l. Inspect catheter integrity and discard.

     ____ ____ ____   _____

Nurse Alert: If catheter is removed for suspected infection, send tip to lab for culturing, along with blood samples.

5. Use Completion Protocol.

     ____ ____ ____   _____

Evaluation

1. Monitor I&O every 8 hours and monitor laboratory values.

2. Evaluate insertion site, catheter/port, and IV system.

     ____ ____ ____   _____

3. Evaluate for complications of therapy.

     ____ ____ ____   _____

4. Monitor vital signs.

     ____ ____ ____   _____

5. Monitor for signs of air embolism and thrombosis.

     ____ ____ ____   _____

- Identify unexpected outcomes and intervene as necessary.

     ____ ____ ____   _____

- Record and report intervention and client's response.

     ____ ____ ____   _____

Performance Checklist: Skill 38.2

Administration of Total Parenteral Nutrition

	S	U	NP	Comments

Assessment

1. Assess indications of and risks for protein-calorie malnutrition. ____ ____ ____ _____

2. Assess serum albumin, total protein, transferrin, prealbumin, triglycerides, glucose, and urine nitrogen balance as ordered by physician. ____ ____ ____ _____

3. Consult with physician and dietitian on calculation of calorie, protein, and fluid requirements for client. ____ ____ ____ _____

4. Assess baseline weight and vital signs. ____ ____ ____ _____

5. Verify physician's order for nutrients, vitamins, minerals, trace elements, electrolytes, and flow rate. ____ ____ ____ _____

Implementation

1. Use Standard Protocol. ____ ____ ____ _____

2. Initiate central line management protocol. ____ ____ ____ _____

3. Explain purpose of total parenteral nutrition (TPN). ____ ____ ____ _____

4. Inspect TPN solution for particulate matter or separation of fat into layer. ____ ____ ____ _____

5. Connect TPN solution to appropriate IV tubing. Prior to connecting TPN solution, flush tubing, then connect to dedicated port of multilumen central catheter, and label port. ____ ____ ____ _____

6. Use IV pump or volume controller to infuse solution. ____ ____ ____ _____

7. Assess appearance of central line site routinely (see agency policy). ____ ____ ____ _____

8. Change tubing every 24 hours or anytime contamination is suspected or integrity of product may have been compromised. ____ ____ ____ _____

9. Discard bag and tubing if contamination of bag or tubing is suspected. ____ ____ ____ _____

	S	U	NP	Comments

10. Do not add medications to parenteral nutrition solution.

11. Make sure adequate solution is available to ensure continuous infusion if ordered.

Nurse Alert: Have backup fluids available if new TPN solution cannot be obtained in time.

12. Use Completion Protocol.

Evaluation

1. Monitor client's weight.

2. Monitor I&O and evaluate for fluid overload or dehydration.

3. Monitor capillary glucose with glucose meter q6h or as ordered.

4. Monitor for signs and symptoms of infection at infusion site.

• Identify unexpected outcomes and intervene as necessary.

• Record and report intervention and client's response.

Performance Checklist: Skill 38.3

Mechanical Ventilation

	S	U	NP	Comments

Assessment

1. Assess the client's level of consciousness and ability and willingness to cooperate or assist with the procedure and the need for special positioning during the intubation procedure. ____ ____ ____ _____

2. Assess the client's ability and willingness to communicate, and establish an appropriate means to do so. ____ ____ ____ _____

3. Assess the client's need for specialized nutrition support. ____ ____ ____ _____

4. Assess the client's baseline vital signs and laboratory values. ____ ____ ____ _____

Implementation

1. Use Standard Protocol. ____ ____ ____ _____

2. Explain the system to the client, using descriptions of anticipated experiences and benefits. ____ ____ ____ _____

3. Set up a communication system and reassure the client that assistance will always be nearby. ____ ____ ____ _____

Nurse Alert: Be sure that communication device or system is always available to client.

4. If client does not have an endotracheal or tracheostomy tube, assist physician with insertion, then order chest x-ray. ____ ____ ____ _____

5. Implement safety and infection-control measures.
   a. Check ventilator and cardiac alarm at the beginning or each shift and after visits to the bedside by others. ____ ____ ____ _____
   b. Check ET tube position in centimeters every shift and secure stabilization of artificial airway with every client contact. ____ ____ ____ _____
   c. Keep airway, face mask, and resuscitation mask at bedside. ____ ____ ____ _____
   d. Ensure availability of emergency supplies on unit. ____ ____ ____ _____

	S	U	NP	Comments

e. Check endotracheal tube cuff using minimal leak technique every shift and after any change in tube position.

f. Verify tube position after every chest x-ray.

g. Using inline catheter, suction prn; suction oropharynx/nasopharynx after endotracheal suctioning and before any cuff manipulation.

h. Use swivel adapter between endotracheal tube and ventilator.

i. Rotate oral endotracheal tube from one side of mouth to the other every 24 hours; retape endotracheal tube every 24 hours and prn, using skin prep pads.

j. Perform oral hygiene every 2 hours.

k. Monitor inline temperature continuously.

l. Keep ventilator tubing clear of condensation and secretions.

m. Place bite block or airway if client is biting tube.

n. Administer sedatives or neuromuscular blocking agents as ordered if client is fighting ventilator and ineffective ventilation occurs; observe carefully after administration.

o. Troubleshoot high-pressure alarms within 15 seconds.

6. Whenever possible, place the client in semi-Fowler's position.

7. If client becomes confused or combative, consult physician on use of soft restraints to prevent the client from extubating self.

8. Monitor arterial blood gases (ABGs) regularly to detect possible overventilation or inadequate alveolar ventilation or atelectasis.
    a. Check oxygen saturation continuously.
    b. Check $EtCO_2$ and SPO_2 levels whenever ventilator settings are changed.
    c. Pulse oximetry and capnography may be used for continuous monitoring of blood gases in addition to periodic laboratory analysis of blood specimens.
    d. Check ABGs whenever a sudden change in client's condition occurs.

9. Perform the following at least hourly:
    a. Make sure that the client can reach the call light if able to use it.
    b. Check all connections between the client and the ventilator, making sure

that the alarms are turned on, including both high- and low-pressure alarms and volume alarms.

c. Verify that the ventilator settings are correct and that the ventilator is operating at those settings. Compare the client's respiratory rate with the settings. Make sure that the spirometer reaches the correct volume for volume-cycled mode; for pressure-cycled machines. Assess exhaled tidal volume.

Nurse Alert: Do not assume that the settings are correct or that the machine is operating correctly.

d. Check the humidifier and refill if necessary. Check the corrugated tubing for condensation, and drain any accumulation to be discarded.

e. Check temperature gauges and make sure that gas is being delivered at the correct temperature (89.6° F [32° C] to 98.6° F [37° C]).

10. At least every 4 hours, assess client for:
a. Confusion, anxiety/restlessness, agitation/lethargy, headache.
b. Adventitious breath sounds, dyspnea, tachypnea, inability to move secretions.
c. Decreased urine.
d. Nasal flaring, tracheal tug, intractable cough, fremitus, use of accessory muscles.
e. Changes in respiratory depth, prolonged expiratory phase, or altered chest excursion during spontaneous breaths.

11. Auscultate for decreased breath sounds on the left side. Arrange for chest x-rays as ordered.

12. Auscultate over trachea for air leaks using stethoscope.
a. Using minimal occlusive pressure, inflate cuff with 10 ml syringe.
b. Leave syringe attached to cuff of tubing.

13. Monitor fluid intake and output (I&O) and electrolyte balance. Weigh client as ordered.

14. Using aseptic technique, change the tubing every 48 hours, including the humidifier, the nebulizer, and the ventilator. During

	S	U	NP	Comments

the tubing change the client should be manually ventilated.

15. Change the client's position frequently.

16. Perform chest physiotherapy as necessary, including percussion and postural drainage as appropriate.

17. Monitor gastrointestinal function to prevent complications.
   a. Administer H_2 blockers and other medications as ordered to reduce gastric acid production.
   b. Auscultate for decreased bowel sounds and check for abdominal distention.
   c. Check nasogastric secretions for blood using Gastroccult or other agency-approved reagent.

18. Provide emotional support to minimize stress. Apprehension and anxiety can increase client's respiratory rate and respiratory effort.
   a. Ensure that means of communication is intact.
   b. Explain procedures and events to client.

19. Maintain activity level at toleration.
   a. Do passive/active range-of-motion (ROM) exercises.
   b. Change position every 2 hours and prn.
   c. Evaluate for rotational therapy.
   d. Assist client to chair two to three times daily if tolerated.
   e. Assist client to stand and walk in place at bedside if tolerated.

20. Initiate interdisciplinary consultations as indicated.

21. Use Completion Protocol.

Evaluation

1. Assess client for secretions and suction as needed.

2. Continuously assess SPO_2 and $EtCO_2$, respiratory status, and vital signs at least every 2 to 4 hours, depending on client's status.

3. Inspect oral and nasal mucosa and lips for integrity and moisture.

4. Monitor daily weights and I&O, and related laboratory values.

	S	U	NP	Comments

5. Use Glasgow Coma Scale to evaluate mental status and level of consciousness. _____ _____ _____ _____

6. Monitor for signs and symptoms of infection. _____ _____ _____ _____

7. Evaluate for signs and symptoms of sleep deprivation. _____ _____ _____ _____

- Identify unexpected outcomes and intervene as necessary. _____ _____ _____ _____

- Record and report intervention and client's response. _____ _____ _____ _____

Performance Checklist: Skill 38.4

Care of the Client Receiving Hemodialysis

	S	U	NP	Comments

Assessment

1. Assess client's weight and compare to weight from end of previous dialysis and dry weight. ____ ____ ____ _____

2. Assess client's vital signs with blood pressure taken in both supine and standing positions. ____ ____ ____ _____

3. Assess client for changes in mentation, speech, and thought processes. ____ ____ ____ _____

4. Assess client's peripheral pulses with special attention to extremity where shunt is located. ____ ____ ____ _____

5. Assess client's heart rate and rhythm. ____ ____ ____ _____

6. Assess client's respiratory rate, rhythm, and quality and character of lung sounds. ____ ____ ____ _____

7. Inspect condition of skin around vascular access. If external device is present, inspect insertion/exit sites. ____ ____ ____ _____

Implementation

1. Use Standard Protocol. ____ ____ ____ _____

2. Thoroughly review steps of procedure with client and family member if new to procedure. If client has received dialysis in the past, ask if there are any questions or if client wants to discuss the experience. ____ ____ ____ _____

3. Restrict fluids to 1000 to 1500 ml/day. ____ ____ ____ _____

4. Develop adequate diet plan in collaboration with dietitian and client. Encourage compliance on the part of the client. ____ ____ ____ _____

5. Before dialysis, provide light meals. ____ ____ ____ _____

6. Routine administration of medications must be altered to avoid complications of dialysis.
   a. Antihypertensives must be withheld in vast majority of clients until after treatment. ____ ____ ____ _____
   b. For IV fluids, lactated Ringer's solution must not be used because of potassium load. ____ ____ ____ _____

c. Calcium for use as a phosphate binder
must be given *with* meal, not just "around
mealtime."

____ ____ ____ _____

7. For care of access:
   a. Palpate for thrill and auscultate for bruit.
   Client should learn to assess bruit/thrill
   daily.

____ ____ ____ _____

   b. If clotting is suspected or confirmed,
   declotting is usually performed in
   radiology.

____ ____ ____ _____

   c. Use dual-lumen catheters for drawing
   blood and giving IV fluids *only* with
   approval of nephrology attending
   physician. Catheter must be flushed with
   heparin after blood is drawn.

____ ____ ____ _____

   d. Post a warning sign in prominent location
   and instruct client to observe by refusing
   to allow others to perform venipuncture
   or blood pressure measurements on
   affected extremity.

____ ____ ____ _____

   e. If access device is external and newly
   placed, clean around insertion site with
   antiseptic swab. Using sterile gloves,
   apply sterile gauze squares or gauze roll
   (see agency policy).

____ ____ ____ _____

8. Use Completion Protocol.

____ ____ ____ _____

Evaluation

1. Compare weight and blood pressure to
preprocedure parameters.

____ ____ ____ _____

2. Ask client to describe general comfort level.

____ ____ ____ _____

3. Observe for nausea, vomiting, change in
vital signs, or altered level of consciousness.

____ ____ ____ _____

4. Palpate arteriovenous shunt for thrill and
auscultate for bruit.

____ ____ ____ _____

5. Ask client to describe the purpose and
process of hemodialysis.

____ ____ ____ _____

• Identify unexpected outcomes and
intervene as necessary.

____ ____ ____ _____

• Record and report intervention and
client's response.

____ ____ ____ _____

Performance Checklist: Skill 38.5

Peritoneal Dialysis

	S	U	NP	Comments

Assessment

1. Assess client's weight and vital signs for baseline. Blood pressure should be measured with the client standing and supine. ____ ____ ____ _____

2. Assess client's serum electrolytes, especially potassium. ____ ____ ____ _____

3. Assess client's knowledge and compliance with diet plan. Review sources of high sodium that often require restriction. ____ ____ ____ _____

Implementation

1. Use Standard Protocol. ____ ____ ____ _____

2. Review client's knowledge of dialysis and provide emotional support. ____ ____ ____ _____

3. Warm dialysate solution to body temperature. ____ ____ ____ _____

4. Add any prescribed medications to dialysate. ____ ____ ____ _____

5. Apply mask and prepare dialysis administration set. Have client wear mask during connection and disconnection of administration set.
   a. Place drainage bag below client. ____ ____ ____ _____
   b. Connect outflow tubing to drainage bag. ____ ____ ____ _____

6. Connect dialysis infusion lines to the bags/bottles of dialysate and hang at client's bedside. ____ ____ ____ _____

7. Place client in supine position when the equipment and solutions are ready. ____ ____ ____ _____

8. Apply gloves. Prime tubing by allowing solution to fill tubes. Keeping clamps closed, connect one infusion line to the abdominal catheter. ____ ____ ____ _____

Nurse Alert: Avoid introducing air into peritoneal cavity.

9. Check patency of catheter.
   a. Rapidly instill 500 ml of dialysate into client's peritoneal cavity. ____ ____ ____ _____

	S	U	NP	Comments

b. Immediately unclamp the outflow line and let fluid drain into the collection bag.

10. Open the clamps on the infusion lines and infuse the prescribed amount of dialysate over 5 to 10 minutes; allow solution to dwell for prescribed interval (10 minutes to 4 hours). Remove and discard gloves and wash hands.

11. When dwell time is completed, open the outflow clamps and allow the solution to drain into the collection bag.

12. Repeat the cycles of infusion-dwell-drainage (using new batches of solution each cycle) until the prescribed amount of dialysate and the prescribed number of cycles have been achieved.

13. When the dialysis treatment is completed, mask the client, put on a mask and sterile gloves, and clamp the catheter.

14. After carefully disconnecting the inflow line from the catheter, place a sterile tip over the catheter end. Discard gloves.

15. Monitor vital signs every 10 minutes, then every 2 to 4 hours.

16. During treatment, have client change positions frequently, do ROM exercises, and do deep breathing.

17. Maintain adequate nutrition, adhering to any prescribed diet.

18. Apply gloves. Maintain standard precautions when emptying collection bag and measuring solution

19. Change dressing every day and prn.
    a. Use Standard Protocol.
    b. Apply gloves. Cleanse insertion site with wound cleanser.
    c. Apply two split-drain sponges around the site and tape securely in place.

20. Use Completion Protocol.

Evaluation

1. Compare weight and blood pressure to preprocedure parameters.

2. Ask client to describe comfort level.

3. Observe for respiratory distress and signs of peritonitis.

	S	U	NP	Comments

4. Observe catheter for patency. Inspect skin condition at catheter site.

5. Ask client to describe the purpose and process of peritoneal dialysis.

- Identify unexpected outcomes and intervene as necessary.

- Record and report intervention and client's response.

Performance Checklist: Skill 39.1

Care of the Dying Client

	S	U	NP	Comments

Assessment

1. Assess each symptom in terms of onset, precipitating factors, quality, severity, and relief measures.

2. Listen for information that indicates spiritual distress on the part of the client or family.

3. Determine barriers to the expression of feelings.

4. Elicit information from client or family that may determine stage of grieving process and coping ability.

Implementation

1. Use Standard Protocol.

2. Promote relief from pain.
   a. Administer appropriate analgesics on an "around the clock" schedule.
   b. Consider the use of adjuvant medication in collaboration with the physician.
   c. Choose the most effective route for analgesics.
   d. Monitor the effectiveness of the medication and adverse side effects.
   e. Monitor for major side effects of narcotic analgesics.
   f. Consider nonpharmacologic methods of pain control.

3. Promote emotional well-being.
   a. Talk with client and family about stressors, anxieties, and fears.
   b. If client is unable to verbalize, observe for signs and symptoms of agitation and emotional distress.
   c. Administer antianxiety medications as indicated and ordered. Observe for signs of depression and need for treatment.
   d. Utilize members of the interdisciplinary team to aid in support.

	S	U	NP	Comments

e. Facilitate communication between client and significant others. ___ ___ ___ _____

f. Involve family in providing care as appropriate. ___ ___ ___ _____

g. Teach family what changes to expect as client's condition worsens. ___ ___ ___ _____

4. Promote spiritual well-being.
   a. Facilitate spiritually meaningful activities. ___ ___ ___ _____
   b. Identify sources of spiritual pain and encourage or seek support for client. ___ ___ ___ _____
   c. Encourage discussion of goals, life review, values, and sense of meaning/hope. ___ ___ ___ _____
   d. Clarify who is handling client's affairs and arrangements to be made. ___ ___ ___ _____

5. Apply gloves. Promote skin integrity and personal hygiene. Reposition frequently. Use pressure-reducing devices. Treat pressure sores. Apply lotion as needed and desired. Provide personal hygiene. ___ ___ ___ _____

6. Promote nutrition as tolerated.
   a. Medicate for nausea and vomiting regularly. ___ ___ ___ _____
   b. Apply gloves. Provide oral hygiene. ___ ___ ___ _____
   c. Offer small amounts of food and fluids of client's preference. ___ ___ ___ _____
   d. Avoid foods with strong odors. ___ ___ ___ _____
   e. Provide information and support to family members. ___ ___ ___ _____

7. Ensure maintenance of elimination.
   a. Regular use of stool softeners and laxatives. ___ ___ ___ _____
   b. Encourage use of bedside commode. ___ ___ ___ _____

8. Promote oxygenation.
   a. Elevate head of the bed. ___ ___ ___ _____
   b. Administer oxygen as ordered. ___ ___ ___ _____
   c. Promote measures to conserve energy. ___ ___ ___ _____
   d. Consider opioid use for severe dyspnea and atropine to decrease secretions. ___ ___ ___ _____

9. Use Completion Protocol. ___ ___ ___ _____

Evaluation

1. Evaluate client's degree of relief from pain and other symptoms. ___ ___ ___ _____

2. Ask about progress in decision making identified by client and family as essential at this time. ___ ___ ___ _____

3. Observe level of participation in care of client, based on wishes of client/family. ___ ___ ___ _____

	S	U	NP	Comments

4. Ask if client/family is satisfied with emotional and spiritual support measures. ____ ____ ____ _____

• Identify unexpected outcomes and intervene as necessary. ____ ____ ____ _____

• Record and report intervention and client's response. ____ ____ ____ _____

Performance Checklist: Skill 39.2

Care of the Body after Death

	S	U	NP	Comments

Assessment

1. Assess for presence of family members or significant others and their knowledge of client's death. Determine who is legally defined as next of kin. ____ ____ ____ _____

2. Assess family's grief response. ____ ____ ____ _____

3. Approach next of kin and for organ/tissue donation. ____ ____ ____ _____

4. Assess client's religious preference and/or cultural heritage. ____ ____ ____ _____

5. Determine whether autopsy is planned. ____ ____ ____ _____

Implementation

1. Use Standard Protocol. ____ ____ ____ _____

2. Assist family to do what they need to do at this time. ____ ____ ____ _____

3. Have body placed in a private room or move roommate. ____ ____ ____ _____

4. Check with significant others about notifying other significant people. ____ ____ ____ _____

5. Discuss procedure of preparing the body with significant others. Inquire if there are particular cultural or spiritual practices that are significant for the deceased or significant others. ____ ____ ____ _____

6. Determine whether family wants to be involved in preparation of body. ____ ____ ____ _____

7. If tissue donation has been made, consult policy for specific guidelines in care of the body. ____ ____ ____ _____

8. Wash hands. Apply gloves or protective barriers as necessary. ____ ____ ____ _____

9. Identify the body according to agency policy. Leave identification in place as directed in agency policy. ____ ____ ____ _____

10. If in keeping with agency procedures, remove all indwelling catheters, IV, oxygen, and other tubes. (If an autopsy is to be performed, policy may direct to leave these devices in place.) Dress puncture wounds with a small dressing and paper tape.

11. Remove soiled dressings and replace with clean gauze dressings. Use paper tape.

12. If the person wore dentures, insert them. If mouth fails to close, place a rolled up towel under the chin.

13. Position client as outlined in agency procedures. In general, do not place one hand on top of the other.

14. Place small pillow or folded towel under the head or elevate head of bed 10 to 15 degrees.

15. Close eyes gently by grasping the eyelashes and pulling the lids over the corneas.

16. Wash body parts soiled by blood, urine, feces, or other drainage. Place an absorbent pad under the client's buttocks.

17. Place a clean gown on the client (agency policy may require removal before body is wrapped).

18. Brush and comb client's hair. Remove any clips, hairpins, or rubber bands.

19. Remove all jewelry and give to family member. EXCEPTION: Family may request wedding band be left in place. Place a small strip of tape around client's finger over the ring.

20. If significant others request viewing, place a sheet or light blanket over the body with only the head and upper shoulders exposed. Remove unneeded equipment from the room. Provide soft lighting and offer chairs. Determine whether they would like a staff member to remain.

21. After the significant others have left the room, remove all linen and the client's gown (refer to agency policy). Place body in body bag or apply the shroud as required by the agency.

22. Label the body as directed by agency policy.

	S	U	NP	Comments

23. Arrange transportation of the body to the morgue or mortuary.

24. Observe the response of significant others and provide an opportunity to express feelings.

25. Use Completion Protocol.

Evaluation

1. Observe significant others' response to loss.

2. Determine whether significant others have received appropriate emotional and spiritual support.

3. Note appearance and condition of client's skin during preparation of body.

• Identify unexpected outcomes and intervene as necessary.

• Record and report intervention and client's response.

Performance Checklist: Skill 40.1

Client Teaching

	S	U	NP	Comments

Assessment

1. Assess client's learning needs and readiness to learn.

2. Assess attention span, short-term memory, pain, fatigue, anxiety level, sensory status, language, and distractions.

3. Assess client's attitudes toward learning and willingness to follow health care provider recommendations.

(4.) Review risk factors from nursing history in relation to lifestyle patterns.

5. Review client's employment history to determine risks in the work setting.

6. Assess client's and family's understanding of therapies, restrictions, and possible complications.

7. Determine client's actual or potential limitations resulting from sensory, motor, cognitive, or physical changes.

8. Consult with other health team members about needs after discharge.

Implementation

1. Use Standard Protocol.

2. Utilize every contact with the client as an opportunity to teach.

3. Together with client and family, identify what the learner needs to accomplish and how achievements will be measured.

4. Select media, methods of teaching, and aids appropriate to client's needs.

5. Establish an environment that encourages client and family to ask questions and participate in decision making and care.

6. When presenting information, vary the tone of voice, use simple, clear language,

	S	U	NP	Comments

and, if possible, reinforce with pictures or demonstrations. Repeat and highlight key points. ___ ___ ___ _____

7. Set up equipment and demonstrate self-care to the client using supplies and equipment that client will be using at home. ___ ___ ___ _____

8. Employ teaching techniques of repetition, rephrasing, and summarizing. ___ ___ ___ _____

9. Have client demonstrate skill. Provide with positive feedback. Have client/family member become as independent as possible with skill. ___ ___ ___ _____

10. Elicit feedback from the client/family frequently. ___ ___ ___ _____

11. Teach health promotional activities as appropriate, including avoidance of risks, safety, screening, nutrition, and exercise. ___ ___ ___ _____

12. As appropriate, teach client how to recognize stress and measures to deal effectively with psychophysiological effects. ___ ___ ___ _____

13. Review material repeatedly as care is provided, asking questions to encourage the client to think about implications for self-care. ___ ___ ___ _____

14. Give client praise for return demonstrations that are done correctly and for behavior changes resulting from information given. ___ ___ ___ _____

15. Use Completion Protocol. ___ ___ ___ _____

Evaluation

1. Evaluate client's and/or caregiver's ability to perform treatments/procedures. ___ ___ ___ _____

2. Ask client to describe strategies for illness prevention or early detection of disease. ___ ___ ___ _____

• Identify unexpected outcomes and intervene as necessary. ___ ___ ___ _____

• Record and report intervention and client's response. ___ ___ ___ _____

Performance Checklist: Procedural Guideline 40-1

Teaching Clients Self-Injections

	S	U	NP	Comments

Implementation

1. Have client hold and manipulate syringe. ____ ____ ____ _____

2. Explain which parts must remain sterile and which can be touched. ____ ____ ____ _____

3. Discuss client's ordered dose. ____ ____ ____ _____

4. Have client check the vial label indicating the type of insulin and expiration date on insulin, and examine solution for color change, clumping, or frosting of the vial. If insulin has been refrigerated, allow to warm to room temperature. ____ ____ ____ _____

5. Have client withdraw medication from vial. Review site selection and rotation. ____ ____ ____ _____

6. Encourage client to insert needle quickly into prepared site all the way to the hub. ____ ____ ____ _____

7. Once needle is inserted, instruct client to slowly let go of skin and transfer free hand to barrel of syringe. ____ ____ ____ _____

8. Have client push plunger all the way in at a slow and steady rate to administer the medication. ____ ____ ____ _____

9. Once medication has been administered, have client quickly remove needle at the same angle it was inserted and exert gentle pressure on the site with a small gauze pad. ____ ____ ____ _____

10. Teach client to dispose of uncapped needle or safety needle in sharps container or hard plastic bottle. Make sure that client is aware of regulations for local sharps disposal. ____ ____ ____ _____

11. Discuss rotation of sites and have client indicate on a chart where the injection was given. ____ ____ ____ _____

12. Encourage client to practice preparing prescribed dose using a bottle of sterile saline. ____ ____ ____ _____

13. Discuss where medication and syringes will be secured at home so that children will not have access to them. ____ ____ ____ _____

Performance Checklist: Skill 40.2

Risk Assessment and Accident Prevention

	S	U	NP	Comments

Assessment

1. Assess client's physical and mental status before discharge and determine the type of adaptations necessary in the home for the client to maintain a healthy state. ___ ___ ___ _____

2. Assess client's attitudes and perceptions toward returning home and following health care provider recommendations. ___ ___ ___ _____

3. Determine client's actual or potential limitations resulting from sensory, motor, cognitive, or physical changes. ___ ___ ___ _____

4. Consult other health team members about needs after discharge. ___ ___ ___ _____

Implementation

1. Use Standard Protocol. ___ ___ ___ _____

2. Prior to discharge, involve client and family as active participants in home safety assessment. ___ ___ ___ _____

3. Identify ways to make home environment safe. ___ ___ ___ _____

4. Reduce the number of different pain medications used. ___ ___ ___ _____

5. Schedule diuretics early in the day. ___ ___ ___ _____

6. Explore benefits and challenges of all recommendations. ___ ___ ___ _____

7. Consider changing the physical environment to reduce predisposition to falls. ___ ___ ___ _____

8. Provide for safe disposal of in-home medical supplies.
   a. Instruct client to place needles, syringes, lancets, or other sharp objects in a hard plastic or metal container such as soda bottles or laundry detergent containers with screw-on or tightly secured lids. ___ ___ ___ _____
   b. Soiled bandages, disposable sheets, and medical gloves are placed in securely

	S	U	NP	Comments

fastened plastic bag before being placed
in garbage can. ___ ___ ___ _____

9. Provide client and family with information
about community health care resources. ___ ___ ___ _____

10. Use Completion Protocol. ___ ___ ___ _____

Evaluation

1. Evaluate client's and/or caregiver's
knowledge of treatment regimen, signs and
symptoms to be reported, and available
community resources. ___ ___ ___ _____

2. Evaluate client's and/or caregiver's ability
to perform treatments/procedures. ___ ___ ___ _____

3. Follow up on an inspection of the home
environment by family/caregiver or home
health nurse. ___ ___ ___ _____

• Identify unexpected outcomes and
intervene as necessary. ___ ___ ___ _____

• Record and report intervention and
client's response. ___ ___ ___ _____

Name _____ Date _____ Instructor's Name _____

Performance Checklist: Skill 40.3

Adapting the Home Setting for Clients with Cognitive Deficits

	S	U	NP	Comments

Assessment

1. Ask client to describe own level of health and how it affects ability to provide self-care. ____ ____ ____ _____

2. Listen carefully to the client. Provide a quiet, well-lit space and avoid interruptions or distractions. Make accommodations for sensory deficits. ____ ____ ____ _____

Implementation

1. Use Standard Protocol. ____ ____ ____ _____

2. Create a list or utilize a calendar for self-care routines if client has difficulty remembering. ____ ____ ____ _____

3. Schedule medications that are likely to cause confusion to be taken at bedtime. ____ ____ ____ _____

4. Space antihypertensives and antiarrhythmic medications at different times to minimize side effects. ____ ____ ____ _____

5. Reduce steps it takes to complete tasks with multiple steps or simplify the task. ____ ____ ____ _____

6. Help client and family develop a schedule for routine daily activities. Post a large calendar for appointments or special events. ____ ____ ____ _____

7. Have caregivers set up activities so that client can complete them, such as dressing. ____ ____ ____ _____

8. Encourage simple and direct communication using a calm and relaxed approach. Use eye contact and touch. Speak in simple words and short sentences. ____ ____ ____ _____

9. Keep clocks, calendars, and personal items throughout rooms where easily seen. ____ ____ ____ _____

10. Routinely remind client of who caregiver is and what the next step will be. ____ ____ ____ _____

11. Facilitate regular naps or rest periods. ____ ____ ____ _____

12. Encourage and support frequent visits by family and friends. Encourage the use of humor and reminiscing. ____ ____ ____ _____

	S	U	NP	Comments

13. Use Completion Protocol. _____ _____ _____ _____

Evaluation

1. Ask client to review the home management activities completed the morning of that day and the day before to determine ability to recall events. _____ _____ _____ _____

2. Ask caregiver to review schedules of daily routines and review approaches used. _____ _____ _____ _____

• Identify unexpected outcomes and intervene as necessary. _____ _____ _____ _____

• Record and report intervention and client's response. _____ _____ _____ _____

Performance Checklist: Skill 40.4

Helping Clients with Self-Medication and Medical Device Safety

	S	U	NP	Comments

Assessment

1. Assess client's cognitive, sensory, and motor function; level of consciousness; sight; hearing; touch; reading ability and comprehension; ability to swallow; ability to ambulate and tolerate activity; and willingness to cooperate.

2. Assess client's medication regimen.

3. Identify where medications are stored in the home.

4. Assess the client's resources to obtain medications when needed.

Implementation

1. Use Standard Protocol.

2. For prescribed medications and over-the-counter medications, schedule and prn, review:
   a. Purpose of medications and their expected effects
   b. How medications work
   c. Dosage schedules and rationale
   d. Common side effects and their relief
   e. What to do if a dose is missed
   f. When to contact the physician

3. Plan for safe administration of medications as scheduled.
   a. Calendars may be made for each week with plastic bags of medications to be taken at specific times.
   b. Egg cartons may be divided into color-coded sections with medications for the day.
   c. Pillboxes may be set up daily or weekly to separate pills into slots for the day of the week and time.
4. Medications should only taken by the person for whom they were prescribed and only as they were prescribed.
5. Monitor expiration dates.

6. Keep medications in the original containers with the label clearly legible. Have pharmacy provide large-print labels, if needed.

7. Remind the client to finish prescribed medications and get refills before the container is empty.

8. Identify appropriate adaptations to facilitate ease and accuracy in administration of nonparenteral medications.

   a. Have medications dispensed by the pharmacist in a container that the client can open easily.

Nurse Alert: Help establish a safe place for medications to reduce risk of accidental ingestion if small children reside in or visit the home.

   b. Use a color-coding system if many medications are prescribed.

9. See Procedural Guideline 40-1 for teaching self-injection technique.

10. Use Completion Protocol.

Evaluation

1. Ask client to state purpose of each medication, side effects, and when to notify physician about problems.

2. Observe client reading each label and ask to explain when each drug should be taken.

3. Observe client's/caregiver's ability to prepare and administer the medications.

4. Ask to see where client/caregiver stores items and observe disposal of medical supplies.

• Identify unexpected outcomes and intervene as necessary.

• Record and report intervention and client's response.

Performance Checklist: Skill 40-5

Using Home Oxygen Therapy

	S	U	NP	Comments

Assessment

1. Assess client's and family's ability to apply and manipulate oxygen equipment while in the hospital or in the home. ____ ____ ____ _____

2. Assess client's and family's ability to determine the signs and symptoms of hypoxia. ____ ____ ____ _____

3. Assess the availability of community resources for home oxygen therapy. ____ ____ ____ _____

4. Assess client's and family's ability to recognize the signs and symptoms of carbon dioxide narcosis. ____ ____ ____ _____

5. Determine appropriate backup system, if compressor is used, in event of power failure. ____ ____ ____ _____

Implementation

1. Use Standard Protocol. ____ ____ ____ _____

2. Place oxygen system in a clutter-free environment. ____ ____ ____ _____

3. Check oxygen level remaining. Maintain a backup supply.
   a. Check liquid system by depressing button at lower right corner and reading the dial on the Liberator or Stroller. ____ ____ ____ _____
   b. Check cylinders by reading amount on pressure gauge. ____ ____ ____ _____

4. Connect oxygen delivery device to oxygen system. ____ ____ ____ _____

5. Determine and set correct liter flow rate. Ensure delivery of prescribed amount of oxygen. ____ ____ ____ _____

Nurse Alert: Equipment vendor and nurse instruct client how frequently Liberator and Stroller must be filled.

6. Review safety guidelines. ____ ____ ____ _____

7. Place oxygen delivery device on client. ____ ____ ____ _____

	S	U	NP	Comments

8. When client is leaving the home and needs portability, the following steps are needed to prepare the portable units.
   a. Verify adequate supply of oxygen in tank by reading gauge on regulator.
   b. Connect appropriate oxygen delivery device and oxygen tubing to Stroller.
   c. Place Stroller on cart.
   d. Set prescribed flow rate and lock flow meter.

9. Use Completion Protocol.

Evaluation

1. Evaluate client's respiratory status and use of oxygen.

2. Ask client and family to describe reasons for and correct setup of home oxygen.

3. Observe client's and/or caregiver's use of home oxygen.

4. Ask client and family to describe safety guidelines.

- Identify unexpected outcomes and intervene as necessary.

- Record and report intervention and client's response.